1 Tablespoon
(basic need)

LECITHIN—THE LIFE YOU SAVE MAY BE YOUR OWN

Atherosclerosis and acne—are usually found in different age groups, but they have one thing in common—the substance that has been shown to have a remarkable effect in alleviating both—lecithin.

Lecithin is a constituent of many foods—though modern processing techniques and dietary practices have drastically cut down the average intake. It is a vital component of the human body. Degenerative and acute conditions too often testify to its absence; but in this authoritative treatment, Carlson Wade explains both our need for lecithin and how we can assure our bodies an adequate supply of it.

A special cookbook section offers tasty recipes employing lecithin in its most readily available forms, for basic sound nutrition, enjoyable eating and special protection against disease and degenerative conditions.

CARLSON WADE'S

Lecithin Book

Keats Publishing, Inc. ● New Canaan, Connecticut

CARLSON WADE'S
LECITHIN BOOK

Copyright © 1980 by Carlson Wade. Special material
Copyright © 1980 by Keats Publishing, Inc.

Printed in the United States of America

Library of Congress Catalog Card Number: 80-82319

PIVOT ORIGINAL HEALTH BOOKS are published by
Keats Publishing, Inc., 36 Grove Street (Box 876)
New Canaan, Connecticut 06840

CONTENTS

INTRODUCTION ....

Chapter 1. Lecithin—How It Can Revitalize
Your Total Health 1

Chapter 2. How Lecithin Can Add Years to
Your Heart 15

Chapter 3. Cleanse Your Arteries and Melt
Cholesterol with Lecithin 25

Chapter 4. The "Dr. Rinse Lecithin Breakfast"
for a Longer Life 39

Chapter 5. How You Can Enjoy Vim-Vigor-Vitality
with Lecithin 53

Chapter 6. How to "Think Young" and Protect
against Senility with Lecithin 63

Chapter 7. Questions and Answers about
Lecithin 77

Chapter 8. Using Lecithin for Beauty 87

Chapter 9. Your Lecithin Cookbook 95

CARLSON WADE'S

LECITHIN BOOK

INTRODUCTION

LECITHIN is being recognized as a powerful total body healer. More and more scientists and researchers in the medical fields are discovering that the use of this all-natural food helps prolong the prime of life, helps protect against so-called "fatal" ailments and gives new hope for better health at almost any age.

This book will show you how lecithin, the miracle food of the century, is able to add years to your heart, cleanse your arteries, and keep cholesterol under control.

A simple "lecithin breakfast" saved a noted scientist's life when he was given just a few years to survive. It is pleasant to eat, easy to prepare and helpful in healing.

A special lecithin cookbook section helps you enjoy this life-saving food in many ways. You can tap your hidden sources of vitality with the use of lecithin. Perhaps the greatest recent discovery is the use of lecithin to activate your sluggish mind and protect you against senility. Lecithin actually helps you "think young" and stay vigorous. You can also use lecithin to improve your skin so that you can look young while you think young.

Lecithin can be your new hope for a life of healthy and happy youthfulness.

CARLSON WADE'S

LECITHIN BOOK

1 LECITHIN—How It Can Revitalize Your Total Health

WAKE UP YOUR BODY! Tap your hidden sources of renewed youth! Energize your thinking powers! Enjoy healthy brain functions! Cleanse your body of age-causing wastes and experience the flow of youthful vitality . . . in a matter of moments. These "make-yourself-over" reactions and many more are possible when you regenerate your body with a little-known but amazingly powerful substance found in a select group of everyday foods. This substance has been hailed as "dynamic" in its powers of self-regeneration for people of almost all ages and under all circumstances. It can help wake up *your* body and *your* mind so that you will look and feel "forever young" and "forever vigorous" for a long, long time.

LECITHIN—THE "TOTAL HEALTH" FACTOR

Lecithin (pronounced *less-i-thin*) is a substance located in almost every one of your trillions of body cells. It is also found in every body organ. It is required by all cells and organs for nourishment and survival. It is as essential to your life as air.

The lecithin you can purchase is a bland, water-

1

soluble granular powder made from de-fatted soybeans. Biochemists call it a *phosphatide*.

The name *lecithin* is taken from the Greek word *likithos* meaning "egg yolk." It is known that egg yolk contains high concentrations of lecithin but also much cholesterol. So if you are on a cholesterol-watching program, egg yolk may not be preferable as your main source of lecithin.

However, lecithin is considered a *phospholipid*, or a fat-melting substance. Therefore, if you eat moderate amounts of egg, you consume both cholesterol and an egg's fat-melting substance, lecithin. Since *both* of these substances are in the egg, it becomes a suitable food as *part* of your healthy diet.

By helping to dissolve fats and cholesterol, lecithin does promote a cleansing reaction within your body. This was noted in *Introduction to Lecithin*, by researcher Howard E. Hill, who points out that lecithin functions as the body's emulsifier. It keeps cholesterol and other fats broken up into microscopic globules which can then freely pass through arterial walls and into your body. So we see that it does constitute a protective factor. The problems of atherosclerosis begin when cholesterol clumps up and adheres to blood vessel walls. These clumps can form fibrous plaques which may grow until they narrow or shut off a vessel. If the closed vessel is one that supplies blood to your heart, the consequence may be a heart attack. But it is lecithin that helps protect against this cholesterol buildup.

TEN HEALTH BENEFITS OF LECITHIN

Research chemist Philip S. Chen, Ph.D., author of *Heart Disease: Cause, Prevention and Recovery* and

Soybeans for Health and a Longer Life notes that "lecithin is a natural product occurring almost universally in the cells of plant and animal life. In the body, the largest amounts are found in the brain and nerve tissues, heart, kidneys and endocrine glands." Dr. Chen then cites these basic ten health benefits of lecithin:

1. *Lowers surface tension.* Lecithin is effective in lowering the surface tension of aqueous solutions. This means lecithin is an effective emulsifying agent, capable of dissolving cholesterol deposits in substances such as the blood. The reason is that one side of the molecule prefers fat, while the other is attracted by water.

2. *Improves absorption.* Lecithin increases the digestibility and absorption of fats because of its emulsifying abilities. It also enhances both the absorption and utilization of vitamin A and carotene (the precursor of vitamin A as obtained from a meatless source). It increases the blood level and storage of vitamin A.

3. *Fat metabolism.* Lecithin boosts the metabolism of fat. The enzyme, *lecithinase*, which is produced in the body, sets choline free to exercise its power to prevent the accumulation of fat in the liver. Choline is able to alter fat into another form, or otherwise remove its accumulation in an organ. Lecithin contains the power to invigorate choline.

4. *Contains lipotropic agents.* Lecithin contains lipotropic agents which are needed to metabolize fats. It contains both choline and inositol (members of the B-complex family) which enter into the fat metabolization process.

5. *Skin health.* Soy lecithin is helpful in treating skin problems such as psoriasis, dry skin, eczema, sclero-

derma, senile atrophy of the skin, seborrhea, acne and keloid formation caused by fat absorption.

6. *Diabetic health.* Lecithin reportedly may be able to decrease the needs of insulin requirements, by assisting better absorption and metabolism of sugars and starches via the pancreas.

7. *Better digestion.* Lecithin improves the absorption of fat and lowers the susceptibility for problems of sprue (improper digestive absorption of fats and carbohydrates) and diarrhea.

8. *Better liver function.* Soy lecithin helps soothe deranged fat metabolism which in turn helps improve problems of liver dysfunction. Dr. Chen says, "lecithin prevents accumulation of fat in the liver, enhances both the absorption and utilization of vitamin A and carotene and increases the blood level and storage of the former."

9. *Kidney health.* Lecithin helps correct deficiencies in choline or other lipotropic agents which may cause hemorrhagic degeneration of the kidney.

10. *Internal cleansing.* The lipotropic substances in soy lecithin often help clear away vitreous opacities (the forerunner of cholesterol deposits—a colorless thickening).

More benefits: Dr. Philip S. Chen refers to published reports in which soy lecithin is found to break up fatty deposits, enabling the entire body to respond with more youthful vigor.

Lecithin can undoubtedly be considered a "youth factor," a regenerator of just about every part of the body and mind.

THE HEALING POWER OF LECITHIN

Many studies have been made of the healing powers of this wonder food. Here is a selection from some clinical reports:

Cholesterol reduction. Lecithin is able to reduce the cholesterol level in the blood. It is also able to break down hard plaques already accumulated and deposited in the arteries. (*Geriatrics,* January 1958.) This is the work of lecithin's ingredient called sitosterol, or soy sterols.

Eases skin discolorations. In doctor-administered amounts, lecithin was able to help ease and eventually erase yellow-brown or yellow blemishes on the skin as well as around the eyes; they were caused by accumulated fatty deposits which lecithin was able to break up, dissolve and eliminate from the body. (*The Low-Fat Way To Health and Longer Life* by Lester M. Morrison, M.D.)

Stimulates resistance to infection. Lecithin increases the supplies of gamma globulin in the bloodstream and this helps build immunity against infectious bacteria. (Drs. Meyer Friedman, Sanford Byers, Ray Rosenman and research associates in San Francisco as quoted by Dr. Morrison in his book.)

Rejuvenates skin. Aging skin can be corrected with supervised amounts of lecithin. Lecithin also helps correct various kinds of blemishes of the skin. (Francis M. Pottenger, Jr., M.D., *Transactions of the American Therapeutic Society,* Volume 43.)

Skin blemishes healed. With the use of simple soy lecithin, skin problems such as acne, eczema and even psoriasis can be cleared up. (*New York Journal of Medicine*, November 15, 1950.)

Important brain stimulant. The use of lecithin is important in helping regenerate and revive sluggish brain cells. Within eight weeks, brain health is regenerated. It is also noted that in unstable persons, there is a corresponding deficiency of lecithin content in the brain. (Raymond Bernard, Ph.D., *The Secret of Rejuvenation.*)

Sexual vigor. From some European countries doctors report that the use of lecithin corrects sexual weakness, glandular exhaustion and nerve disorders. It is noted that male reproductive fluid is high in lecithin; therefore, say researchers, if it is deficient, then the sexual powers of virility are simultaneously diminished. (Dr. Bernard, as above.)

In *Heart Disease*, Dr. Chen says that testosterone, the male sex hormone, is prepared from sitosterol: "the hormone promotes growth and normal functioning of the accessory male sex organs and the development of secondary male sex characteristics."

Special help for women. According to Dr. Chen, the sitosterol or soy sterols found in lecithin helps prevent "spontaneous abortion in pregnant women and undue menstrual pain in non-pregnant women.

Use in rheumatoid arthritis. Cortisone, often used to ease the pain of rheumatoid arthritis, is made from soybean sterols.

These and many more reports appear regularly on the youth-creating powers of lecithin.

LECITHIN—WHAT'S IN IT FOR YOU?

To begin, soy lecithin is considered an excellent source of this substance. You can enjoy soybeans which, of course, contain lecithin. And, you can try *soy lecithin granules* (available at all health stores) for a highly concentrated source of this life-building substance. Now, when you take soy lecithin granules, what do they offer? Here's a chart telling you just what's in lecithin for you.

NUTRITIVE CONTENTS OF LECITHIN
100 grams or about 3½ ounces or 7 tablespoons

Moisture (%)	1.33 grams
Protein (%)	4.53 grams
Fiber	Trace amounts
Calcium	92 milligrams
Phosphorus	2140 milligrams
Copper	100 micrograms
Iron	6.5 milligrams
Magnesium	164 milligrams
Potassium	170 milligrams
Vitamin A	100 units
Thiamine	11.5 grams
Riboflavin	33 grams
Pantothenic acid	5.59 grams
Niacin	12 grams
Pyridoxine	29 grams
Choline	2.931 grams
Vitamin K	589 units
Inositol	2.1 grams
Folic acid 60 grams	

(Source: A. E. Staley Mfg. Co., Decatur, Illinois.)

WHAT FORM OF LECITHIN SHOULD YOU USE?

Lecithin is available in liquid, powder and granule form. But it is the *granule* form that is used more frequently in medical programs and therefore this would appear to be most beneficial.

Use lecithin by sprinkling several teaspoons in soups or over salads, blend it with beverages, use it in baked goods and with fruit or vegetable juices. It is great with cereals, cold or hot. Try it with yogurt or dairy dishes, too. Take advantage of lecithin's emulsifying abilities by adding the granules to gravies, sauces and dressings.

NUTRITIVE CONTENTS PER SERVING OF LECITHIN

One tablespoon (7.5 grams) of pure lecithin granules contains:

Calories	51
Carbohydrates	1 gram
Fat (90% of calories)	6 grams
Polyunsaturated fatty acids	3 grams
Mono-saturated fatty acids	1 gram
Saturated fatty acids	1 gram
Cholesterol	0
Choline	250 milligrams
Inositol	250 milligrams
Phosphorus	225 milligrams
Potassium	165 milligrams
Linoleic Acid	3225 milligrams
Linolenic Acid	300 milligrams

NOTE: Since it contains extremely small amounts of naturally present sodium (less than 0.003 grams per serving), lecithin granules may be used freely by those on low-sodium diets.

Even small amounts of lecithin can improve the workability of the batter of any baking mixture and improve the quality of the finished product.

Because of its ability to protect fats and oils from becoming rancid, lecithin naturally preserves freshness, protects the fat-soluble vitamins from oxidation, and promotes better digestion of the fats used in the mixture.

One level tablespoon is generally considered an average daily serving, since that quantity (about 7.5 grams) will provide substantial amounts of high-quality lecithin. If you feel your body requires more, you may safely eat several tablespoons daily. Its effect is characterized by renewed vigor of body and thought processes, as will be detailed in Chapters 5 and 6. Remember, it is a *food* and you can enjoy as much as you desire.

What about liquid lecithin?

This is a semi-concentrated product. Unlike the oil-free granules, the liquid contains more than 35 percent oil. This is a sticky, not too tasty substance but it is economical as compared with the more potent granules. It is considered to be of lower quality than the granules.

What about lecithin capsules?

A lecithin capsule eliminates the liquid's unpleasant taste and consistency, but it supplies only small quantities of lecithin. Since more than one-third of the contents of a capsule is oil, then the capsules are a high-calorie, *low potency*, uneconomical means of lecithin supplementation. It would take about ten 1200 milligram capsules, the largest capsule available, to supply as much soy phosphatides as one tablespoon (7.5 grams) of lecithin granules.

What about imitation lecithin?

There is an *imitation* version of lecithin granules on the market. Unfortunately, the word "imitation" does not always appear on the label. The ingredients listed do, however, reveal that this product is predominantly soy flour and other inexpensive powders which are added to the liquid grade of lecithin. Far from being a concentrated source of lecithin, the small diluted amount used here provides only a fraction of the phosphatides present in true lecithin granules. So: To be assured of the highest quality lecithin, *read the label*. As a source of lecithin, the soybean is without equal. A pure product will contain nothing but soybean lecithin granules.

Advantages of natural lecithin

Scientists report that the naturally derived product has more effective healing powers than the synthetic variety. This can be more readily understood when we see that there *is* a difference between natural and synthetic lecithin.

In natural soybean lecithin, substances such as choline and inositol are bonded with phosphorus and form what we identify as a *phosphatide*. During the metabolic process, both choline and inositol disengage themselves from the bond and create internal and external regeneration. At the same time, the "liberated" phosphorus is able to nourish and rejuvenate the body skeletal structure, revive brain and nerve tissue, and enter into renewed construction. This is possible when you take natural lecithin containing the *phosphatide* connection.

Why granules are preferable

Phosphatides or phospholipids are molecules that contain the essential polyunsaturated fatty acids and the nutrients listed in the preceding chart. The *quality* and *quantity* of phosphatides in lecithin will determine its health-building values. In lecithin granules, the phosphatide potency appears to be at its highest level and therefore this form is the most effective.

Regulations require pure lecithin granules to have a minimum of 90 percent soy phosphatides. The product label will usually say that it contains *phosphatidyl choline* and this gives assurance that it is a healthful product to use. The *higher* the percentage of *phosphatidyl choline*, the more potent the lecithin.

Most commercial lecithin is prepared from the soybean, considered a superior source of this substance. Soybean oil contains most of the lecithin. By removing almost all of the oil, it is then possible to create pure lecithin granules. Some 1000 pounds of soybeans are needed to create 3 pounds of pure lecithin granules. These are easy to digest, convenient to use, pleasant to taste and offer the highest source of natural soybean phosphatides.

YOU CAN *SEE* LECITHIN AT WORK

When you roast a fatty cut of meat, let the juices collect in a pan and cool off. Note that the fatty globules rise to the top. Now sprinkle a tablespoon of lecithin on top of the fat. Shortly, you'll discover that the fat has disappeared. The juices are there, but where is the fat? Simple. The lecithin had emulsified the fat so that it can be easily disposed of. The same happens when you eat a fatty meal and include lecithin as a supplement. It helps break up the fatty deposits so they have less accumulative power.

YOU CAN *FEEL* LECITHIN AT WORK

In your *brain*, lecithin choline will be transformed into *acetylcholine*, a substance that is able to relay information from one nerve cell to another. This helps emotional reflexes gain strength and vigor.

In your *liver*, lecithin metabolizes fat. There is less chance of liver degeneration.

In your *bloodstream*, lecithin acts as a "guard" in preventing fat from accumulating on the walls of your arteries.

In your *intestinal tract*, lecithin will help the absorption of the skin- and bone-rebuilding vitamins, A and D, and influence the utilization of the other fat-soluble nutrients such as vitamins E and K.

By taking lecithin as a supplement in granule form, or eating foods containing lecithin, you will actually *feel* this substance improving the health of your internal organs.

WHERE TO FIND LECITHIN IN FOODS

Lecithin is in egg yolk and organ meats such as liver, brain, kidneys and heart. Soybeans are regarded as the most potent source. Lecithin is also found in oil-bearing seeds. It is found in wheat as well as in milk.

Does this mean that if you eat a variety and an abundance of these foods, you'll be lecithin-nourishing your body to a satisfactory level? Unfortunately, this seems difficult. You would have to eat a great many egg yolks daily to provide enough lecithin, but this might also provide too much cholesterol to deal with. As for the other foods, they are healthful but they have been processed—and this causes lecithin loss. Milk is pasteurized, wheat is milled, vegetable oils are refined. Organ meats may have more calories and saturated fat than you would desire. So while these are good foods, they should not be looked upon as the sole source of your lecithin. Instead, the use of lecithin granules as a supplement would make up for that which is lost in processing of foods.

Soybean lecithin has unique power

In his classic work, *Soybeans for Health and a Longer Life*, Dr. Chen tells us,

"The phosphatide or lecithin (including cephalin and inositol) content of the soybean is over 3 percent. *This amount is MORE than that found in any other plant and is equal to that found in eggs*. The lecithin in the soybean is identical with that in egg yolk.

"Lecithin is an important constituent of all organs of the human body and especially of the nervous tissue, the heart and the liver. [It has been found that the percentage of lecithin in these organs rises while on a soybean diet. The soybean, therefore, is a good nerve and brain food.] It has thus been used, namely, in preparations for the cure of nervous diseases."

Use soybeans as part of your total health program

While lecithin granules (the natural variety) are powerhouses of important phosphatides, the use of soybeans in everyday eating will nourish your body and provide a good source of essential nutrients. Soybeans contain lecithin and by eating them, you get this vital substance, first hand.

Try some of these soybean foods:

- Canned green soybeans are usually available all seasons.
- Fresh green soybeans are in the market in late Summer or Fall and make a succulent lecithin-rich vegetable. Use them in favorite recipes in place of lima beans.
- Dried soybeans may be purchased the year around and are prepared for eating in the same ways as other dried beans.
- Soybean sprouts may be purchased or grown at home. They make a tasty lecithin-high addition to salads and can also be served as a vegetable.
- Soybean milk, prepared from dry soybeans, may replace cow's milk in most recipes and can be used as a beverage, by itself.
- Soybean mash or pulp is the solid material left after soybean milk is prepared. A great lecithin source.
- Soybean curd is prepared from soy milk and may be purchased fresh, canned or as an instant powder.
- Soy sauce, a fermented product made from soybeans, is used as a seasoning, especially in Oriental foods.
- Soybeans are also available in the form of cold-pressed oils, flour and grits.

Recipe suggestions covering a variety of courses are found in Chapter 9, "Your Lecithin Cookbook."

However you prepare it, lecithin is considered a "wonder food" in the search for a natural way to stimulate the rejuvenation of body and mind.

2 How Lecithin Can Add Years to Your Heart

SEVENTY-TWO TIMES a minute, more than 100,000 times a day, your heart beats to keep the five or six quarts of blood in your cardiovascular system moving. That means moving more than 18,000,000 barrels of blood in a seventy-year life span.

The continuous cardiovascular process

The system involves the pump (heart muscle), the pipes (in particular, the arteries) and the fluid that flows through the system (blood).

Heart valves close as the muscle contracts, relaxes, rests and beats again, each time sending two ounces of blood, laden with oxygen and other nutrients needed by your body's cells, bursting into the circulation at more than a foot a second.

Flowing first through smooth-walled, pencil-thick, expandable arteries that branch and branch again into smaller and more numerous vessels, the blood eventually winds its way into millions of tiny capillaries so narrow that cells can only trickle through them in single file.

Oxygen and nutrients are exchanged for carbon dioxide and cells wastes through the capillary walls. Now the trip back to the heart begins. Blood passes through ever larger and larger veins at one-third the speed with which it began its journey. Eventually, it reaches the heart, is pumped out into the lungs to exchange its carbon dioxide for a fresh supply of oxygen, and returns to the heart to start the cycle over again.

This process should continue for more than seventy years. It should continue for 100 years, and even longer. But there are mishaps. The cardiovascular system becomes abused or "choked" so that the rhythm is delayed or halted. This results in premature illness (it can begin as early as infancy) and a shortened lifespan. Does this have to happen? Cannot the heart continue on and on and on? What goes wrong?

When something goes wrong

The heart may be weakened by disease developing from outside or inside the system which slows both the pumping action and the blood flow. The volume of blood in the system may be increased (by sodium, for example) and strain the heart. The blood pressure may be so great over a long period that the pliable arterial walls have no chance to relax and gradually lose their elasticity. Stiffened, they are unable to accommodate the demands of strenuous activity and may rupture.

Clogged arteries. Most of the time, however, what happens is that the inner walls of arteries thicken as a variety of materials are deposited in and on them; this continues until the buildup blocks the flow of blood entirely. Or until a portion of one deposit breaks loose from the wall, floats by and lodges in the space narrowed by another, similarly cutting off the blood flow.

Blood must keep moving. When the flow is stopped and parts of the body are cut off from their supply of oxygen and nutrients, they begin to die. Brain tissue can survive for only four minutes without blood; heart muscle for twenty to forty minutes. No cells can exist an hour without this blood supply.

The results are known by a variety of names— *myocardial infarction* (damage to the heart muscle that produces the classical "coronary" or "heart attack"), *stroke* (interference with blood supply to the brain), *cerebral hemorrhage* (bleeding from a burst artery to the brain), *peripheral vascular disease* (reduction in blood supply to smaller blood vessels, distant from the heart, which often leads to gangrene), *ischemia* (reduced blood supply to the heart or other organ), *angina pectoris* (chest pains produced by ischemia and worsened by emotional stress or physical exertion), which can lead to serious and sometimes fatal *tachycardia* (very rapid heart beat) and *fibrillation* (chaotic, disorganized heart action). All are products of the vascular disease process.

THE SLOW PROCESS OF ARTERIOSCLEROSIS

Underlying most of the preceding difficulties is the slow, but often steady, process of *arteriosclerosis*—the narrowing and hardening of arteries that make them lose their flexibility. The basic type of this ailment is *atherosclerosis*—that buildup of plaque in arterial walls that narrows an artery, often until it is blocked in one of several ways as described above. Then, an occlusion (a cutting off of blood flow) occurs. All during the progress of arteriosclerosis the heart is unable to function efficiently and the process of body aging is underway. This may well be the root cause of premature fatalities. Does this have to be? Not so, when scientists have found that there is a natural food that is able to nourish and protect the heart.

Clean arteries + low cholesterol = heart health

Doctors and scientists say that one way to keep your heart healthy is keeping your arteries clean and your cholesterol down to a safe level. To keep your blood vessels "open" you need to follow a low animal fat diet, reduce (or eliminate) refined sugars and starches and also avoid salt in all its forms. Physical exercise, too, is part of the program towards maintaining healthy arteries. But you can do more than keep your arteries clean. You can help *counteract* and *correct* the potential harm done by accumulated deposits on your arteries. The extremely effective approach includes the use of lecithin.

Lecithin—the heart cleanser

Two physicians, Charles E. Butterworth, Jr., M.D. and Carlos Krumdieck, M.D., with the Nutrition Program of the School of Medicine of the University of Alabama in Birmingham, report that lecithin has an amazing heart-cleansing effect. Writing in the *American Journal of Clinical Nutrition* (August 1974), the doctors tell us one basic fact about lecithin:

The body requires an enzyme called *lecithin cholesterol acyltransferase* (LCAT) in order to control the buildup of cholesterol on the walls of the arteries. The doctors say that in order for the body to make self-protecting LCAT, it requires lecithin.

There *are* differences among the sources of lecithin. Drs. Butterworth and Krumdieck tell of tests in which animals were given lecithin from an egg yolk (saturated lecithin); it was not too effective in scrubbing away accumulated cholesterol from heart-artery walls. But when the doctors used *polyunsaturated lecithin* from a soybean source, there was a much greater effectiveness in cleansing the heart.

Furthermore, the doctors say that there is "some intriguing preliminary evidence" that people who have had heart attacks or suffer from serious disease of the coronary arteries "have unusually low levels of the lecithin-rich LCAT enzyme." This suggests that the use of lecithin on a daily basis (from a soybean source, preferably in the form of granules) would do much to create "health insurance" for the heart and protection against cholesterol buildup.

HOW LECITHIN SAVED LIVES

David Adlersberg, M.D., and Harry Sobotka, Ph.D., report treating a number of heart-troubled individuals with high cholesterol levels. Writing in the *Journal of the Mt. Sinai Hospital* (Vol. 9, pp. 955-56), the doctors describe how "a striking decrease of the serum cholesterol was achieved by addition of commercial lecithin in the diet."

At age fifty-five, one woman was a diabetic, and overweight. She was given 15 grams of soybean lecithin a day (about two tablespoons of lecithin granules). At the start, she had a cholesterol reading of 360. Six weeks on the daily lecithin program reduced the cholesterol to 235. Still too high, but no longer dangerous. Drs. Adlersberg and Sobotka then took her off the lecithin. Her cholesterol zoomed upward again, proving that lecithin could provide the needed cholesterol reduction.

Another woman aged forty-one had a cholesterol reading dangerously high at 620. The doctors gave her 12 grams of soybean lecithin daily. Two months later, the count was 420. One month after that, it was reduced to 300. Lecithin was correcting her cholesterol and protecting her heart.

A thirty-five-year old man had a 440 cholesterol count that dropped to 260 within eight weeks on a daily dosage of 12 grams of lecithin granules.

Aged thirty-eight, a woman had an extremely dangerous cholesterol reading of 1370 and showed fatty plaques on her skin. She was given 15 grams of lecithin a day. Within ninety days, her cholesterol reading dropped to 445, still dangerously high but with hope for her survival. Her skin condition cleared up, too.

, Drs. Adlersberg and Sobotka believe that with the use of lecithin these patients had been given new hope for longer lives, thanks to cleaner arteries and a healthier heart.

Helps reduce dangerous blood fat

As stated earlier, high amounts of fat circulating in the blood can actually "choke" the heart and restrict its life-giving function. Therefore, doctors feel that if lecithin could combat this problem, the heart would be able to work efficiently.

In *Medical World News* (November 22, 1974), it was reported that physicians with the Simon Stevin Research Institute in Bruges, Belgium, treated 100 patients who were diagnosed as having type II hyperbetalipoproteinemia (excessive levels of blood fat).

The doctors gave them lecithin injections for fourteen days. The results were that those they treated experienced a welcome reduction in blood fat (especially excess plasma cholesterol, which was diminished by 40 percent.

Furthermore, the Institute's director, Dr. Hubert H. Peeters, says that lecithin "is a nontoxic, natural product with no local reactions and no side effects observed in the organs. It can be in the stomach for a long time and present no problems, regardless of age and sex."

Injection or supplements? There is a difference because oral supplements produced "results similar to those obtained after the intravenous therapy, though not to the same degree." Even so, supplements were effective, and are advised for problems of blood fat excesses.

THE DOCTOR PRESCRIBES: LECITHIN SUPPLEMENTS

A noted Los Angeles physician, Lester M. Morrison, M.D., is considered a pioneer in the use of lecithin supplements for cholesterol control and heart improvement.

It was Dr. Morrison who noted that a low-fat diet would do much to help control and even prevent atherosclerosis and subsequent heart distress. But in *Geriatrics* (January 1958) he made this discovery:

A low-fat diet was helpful but in his patients, it did not satisfactorily reduce serum cholesterol of his patients *until lecithin was added to the regimen.*

Furthermore, several of his patients had a history of angina pains but after taking lecithin for three months, "all symptoms of angina pectoris disappeared . . ."

Some twelve out of his fifteen patients who were prescribed soybean lecithin supplements enjoyed an average drop of serum cholesterol of 156 milligrams or 41 percent after three months of this lecithin program. Dr. Morrison again emphasizes that it was the *lecithin* that produced this desirable drop. Without lecithin, results were negligible.

In the beginning, 36 grams (about six tablespoons of lecithin granules) were prescribed for daily use. Dr. Morrison says that a maintenance dose of just one or two tablespoons of lecithin daily (6 to 12 grams) could help control and sustain normal levels of cholesterol.

It seems that a low-fat diet is helpful but it is lecithin that acts as the fat emulsifier and the spark plug to ignite fat metabolism.

LECITHIN CONTROLS HDL-LDL LEVELS

Lecithin, it appears, is able to help promote the increase of high-density lipoproteins (HDLs) and reduction of low-density lipoproteins (LDLs).

High-density lipoproteins are substances in the body that tend to hasten the removal of free cholesterol from the cells (including arterial smooth-muscle cells) to the liver for eventual excretion. Low-density liproproteins are too weak to do this job and may even displace the HDLs so that this cleansing action is reduced. LDLs, on the other hand, can carry cholesterol from the liver to the tissues and are associated with the development of atherosclerosis. Therefore, your goal is to have a *high* level of HDL as compared to a lower level of LDLs.

Lecithin, with its high choline and inositol factors, appears to help bring about an increase in the manufacture of HDLs needed to control your cholesterol deposits and protect your heart from the threat of being choked off. Lecithin is able to invigorate the HDLs to act as an intracellular "bouncer" thereby displacing and discharging undesirable cholesterol and fatty plaque buildup. In addition to controlling your weight, having regular exercise, avoiding the use of tobacco and alcohol, you need to boost your intake of lecithin for a healthy cardio-vascular system.

MAKING THE LECITHIN CONNECTION

Cholesterol is transported through the blood as part of larger molecules known as lipoproteins, consisting of fat, protein, cholesterol and lecithin. As has been noted, your risk of heart trouble may be related to the levels of HDLs in your bloodstream.

In order for cholesterol to be mobilized or moved around your body properly, *it must be hooked up with lecithin from a plant source*. You could obtain your lecithin from such sources as egg yolk, dairy products, organ meats, some authorities believe, but you would be adding fat to your fire, so to speak. Instead, you could use a *cholesterol-free* source of lecithin. Namely that of the soybean. Furthermore, soybean lecithin is rich in polyunsaturated fatty acids which help break down accumulations and keep your heart sparkling clean. When looking for a way to raise your HDL levels, look to soybean lecithin as a powerful source.

AFTER A CORONARY

In his publication, *Lecithin and Health*, Edward R. Hewitt tells us:

"Coronary thrombosis is due to cholesterol deposits in the arteries which finally interfere with the blood supply passing through the heart.

"After a patient has survived a coronary attack and is better, if he takes an ample amount of lecithin continually, the injurious cholesterol deposits will be gradually removed and there will be no more coronary attacks.

"Such a person should take lecithin regularly for the rest of his life, and he will probably have no further attacks.

"I have seen numbers of such cases, and they all do well unless severe damage has been done to the heart organ.

"There is a well known doctor in Florida who has treated over sixty cases of coronary thrombosis in this way, and reports that they are all doing well and none of them has died, so that he can get no sections of their arteries for examination. He says that his patients may all outlive him as he is now over seventy."

Therefore, even after a coronary, lecithin would appear to be beneficial.

There is no need to run the risk of heart trouble. It would be unwise to look away from this potential heart- and life-saving food. Take care of your heart while it is still healthy.

3 Cleanse Your Arteries and Melt Cholesterol with Lecithin

CHOLESTEROL is an emotional word. It conjures up visions of artery-burdened circulation and a choking heart. Yet, cholesterol is an important and even *essential* component of your body. The problem is that you may have too much cholesterol and this could be a risk. Let's take a closer look at this substance.

What is cholesterol? A fat-like substance found in almost all body tissues. It is a component of brain and nerve cells. It is required for the manufacture of various sex hormones such as estrogen in the female. Cholesterol is needed to maintain the structural integrity of your cells. It is required for blood clotting, to insulate nerve fibers and to nourish your brain. As a structural element, cholesterol is found in all cell membranes and the sheaths around certain nerve fibers called myelin sheaths. If cholesterol performs so many vital functions, why the feeling of fright at the mention of the word?

Too much of a good thing. Cholesterol is not all that bad but an *overload* of this substance can give you too much of a good thing. It can cause hypercholesterolemia (excessive blood cholesterol) and this is a serious risk factor. Since this fat-like substance is a main ingredient in the lining of arteries, too much can cause accumulation and this may "choke" the arteries and predispose to arteriosclerosis or hardening of the arteries.

To put it simply, cholesterol is necessary for optimal body functioning. But you don't want it to lie around inert in large hunks choking up your arteries.

How can you keep your cholesterol levels from becoming undesirably high?

Since many scientists believe that dietary cholesterol can contribute to atherosclerosis, cut down on animal foods. (Cholesterol is NOT found in plant foods, just animal foods.) Exercise regularly. Give up smoking and drinking. All this can be of help. But remember, your body manufactures cholesterol and even on an all vegetarian diet, you could have high levels. The answer seems to be in some mechanism whereby excessive cholesterol would be liquefied and discharged. This may well be the most important part of your basic program. How can this be accomplished? The answer is: *lecithin.*

THE CHOLESTEROL-MELTING POWERS OF LECITHIN

In *Let's Eat Right To Keep Fit*, the noted nutrition researcher, Adelle Davis, writes:

"Another cousin of the fat family, lecithin is supplied by all natural oils. . . . Lecithin is an excellent source of the two B vitamins, choline and inositol. If health is to be maintained, the more fat eaten, the larger must be the intake of these two vitamins.

"This substance (lecithin) can be made in the intestinal wall provided choline, inositol and essential fatty acids are supplied.

"Lecithin appears to be a homogenizing agent, capable of breaking fat and probably cholesterol into tiny particles which can pass readily into the tissues. There is evidence that coronary occlusion is associated with deficiencies of linoleic acid and the two B vitamins, choline and inositol, and perhaps with a lack of lecithin itself.

"Huge particles of cholesterol get stuck in the walls of the arteries; they might be homogenized into tiny particles if sufficient nutrients were available for the normal production of lecithin. When oils are refined or hydrogenated, lecithin is discarded!"

This emphasizes the importance of pure and unrefined or non-hydrogenated oils. Use these. They contain appreciable amounts of lecithin that you need for cholesterol control.

How lecithin helps unlock fats and keep them moving

Adelle Davis further cheers lecithin in *Let's Get Well* by explaining how it aids in the transportation of fats: it helps the cells to remove fats and cholesterol from the blood and to utilize them. This action further boosts the production of bile acids made from cholesterol, thereby reducing the amount in the blood.

"Lecithin is a powerful emulsifying agent and for this very reason is particularly important in preventing and correcting atherosclerosis.

"Although blood is essentially water into which fats cannot dissolve, lecithin, if present in normal amounts, causes cholesterol and neutral fats to be broken into microscopic particles which can be held in suspension, pass readily through arterial walls, and be utilized by the tissues."

She shows how lecithin is able to flow directly into the arteries and change blood fat particles from large to small size so that they can then pass through the arterial walls. Its value as a cholesterol-controller cannot be underestimated.

Lecithin keeps your arteries clean

Phospholipids, a publication of the American Lecithin Company, tells us:

"Cholesterol in the bloodstream does not in itself cause atherosclerosis. It is not until it has been precipitated out of the bloodstream upon the arterial surface, whether from chylemicrons or from giant molecules, that it can act to produce characteristic atheromatic lesions. This precipitation is due to disturbance of the delicate balance necessary for the maintenance of colloidal stability.

"Fat and cholesterol *per se* are insoluble in water and equally in blood plasma. A lipid particle containing fat or cholesterol is maintained in colloidal dispersion in the plasma by means of stabilizing, solubilizing, or emulsifying agents.

"In order to be an effective stabilizing or solubilizing agent, a compound must have both fat-soluble and water-soluble groups. The simple explanation usually given for this type of emulsification is that the fat-soluble groups are anchored in the fatty substrate of the particle with the water-soluble polar groups extending out into the aqueous medium. Soy lecithin has been well known for many years to be a very effective emulsifying and solubilizing agent for lipids.

"In the bloodstream, also, it has been believed for many years that lecithin and other phospholipids act in a similar manner, along with other emulsifying or hydrotropic agents. These include the proteins, and to a lesser extent, cholesterol esters.

"It is not difficult to believe that the concentration of lecithin and other phospholipids or, more appropriately, the ratio of phospholipid: cholesterol or phospholipid: total lipid (cholesterol plus fat) may be significant in maintaining stable colloidal dispersion.

"Thus, for example, with a given physical stress, such as vibration, an unstable lipid dispersion may be precipitated, while a relatively more highly solubilized or stable dispersion will not be precipitated.

"In coronary thrombosis, both phospholipids and cholesterol increase in the patient, but cholesterol rises at a more rapid rate than the phospholipids.

"As the phospholipids (in lecithin) are believed to be the controlling factor in keeping the cholesterol dissolved in the blood, the importance of influencing the disturbed balance is stressed. It can be achieved by either reducing cholesterol without lowering the phospholipid content of the blood, or, in reverse, elevation of phospholipids and maintenance of the cholesterol at a constant level."

The phosphatides of soybeans contain lecithin and this is a prime source of *unsaturated* fatty acids which can cause the needed break up of accumulated cholesterol deposits.

THE DOCTOR WHO RECOMMENDS LECITHIN

We have cited the findings of Lester M. Morrison, M.D., author of *The Low Fat Way To Health and Longer*

Life. He feels that with a doctor-supervised program, it is possible to control cholesterol with lecithin. He says that lecithin is able to dissolve and remove atherosclerotic plaques from the bloodstream.

. Dr. Morrison explains how this happens: "In the course of our research, we have found that lecithin apparently has the ability to increase the cholesterol esterases in the human bloodstream. These esterases are enzymes or activators, that aid in the metabolizing of fats."

Dr. Morrison tells us that patients who followed his prescribed lecithin program experienced a sense of well-being. "They said they had more vitality, did not grow tired so quickly as they had formerly, and were in better health than before." He emphasizes that "lecithin is one of our most powerful weapons against disease. It is an especially valuable bulwark against development of hardening of the arteries and all the complications of heart, brain and kidney that follow.

The Doctor's basic program

Dr. Lester M. Morrison suggests the use of a doctor-supervised supplement program. He offers this five-step program to his patients:

1. Include daily, as a food supplement at breakfast, two to four tablespoonfuls of lecithin granules.
2. Each day take B-complex vitamins in the most potent form. Avoid the cheaper preparations which provide only small and ineffectual quantities of the vitamins and have little or no effect on your body.
3. Add to the daily diet at least 25,000 units of vitamin A and 150 milligrams of vitamin C.

4. Take two tablespoons of soybean oil, corn oil or safflower oil daily to provide the essential fatty acids necessary to proper nutrition. The oil may be used as a salad dressing, taken with tomato or fruit juice, or in any way you prefer.

5. Include in your diet two to four tablespoons of whole wheat germ each day. This may be eaten as a breakfast cereal with fruit, or sprinkled in your salad.

Case histories cited by Dr. Morrison

Skin cleared up. A forty-five-year old housewife had fat plaques of yellowish hue on her skin. Following the doctor's lecithin program, the patches vanished entirely. The same "washing" of fat occurred within her arteries.

Chest pains stopped. A forty-five-year old baker was troubled with chest pains (called angina, caused by an interference in the blood supply to the heart muscle). The man could not work. He had yellowish-brown plaques under his eyes. His cholesterol level was "high in the abnormal range." Dr. Morrison prescribed a low-cholesterol and low-fat diet. He also gave him lecithin and high potency vitamins. Within a few months, the chest pains were gone. His cholesterol level was lowered appreciably. The fatty plaques (xanthalasma) vanished from his face. Soon he had been healed.

Conclusions: In extolling the miracle benefits of lecithin, Dr. Morrison says, "After more than ten years of intense experimentation, not only with lecithin, but with a large number of other cholesterol-reducing preparations used in the treatment of heart disease, atherosclerosis and allied conditions, *we found lecithin to give the most rewarding result*. In fact, it was not only useful in treatment of heart and blood vessel disease, *but also in their prevention.*"

Maintaining blood balance

A rule-of-thumb guideline is set by Dr. Roger J. Williams in *Nutrition Against Disease.* This world-famous biochemist says:

"A better answer to the problem of cholesterol deposits might be this: 'Consume more lecithin.' It is known that lecithin has soap-like characteristics, is a powerful emulsifying agent, and its presence in the blood tends to dissolve cholesterol deposits.

"When there is substantially more lecithin in the blood than cholesterol—a ratio of 1.2 to 1 is said to be favorable—the actual amount of cholesterol can be high without the blood plasma getting milky or showing a tendency to produce fatty deposits.

"Lecithin is an enemy of cholesterol deposits and consuming more lecithin is a useful preventive measure."

Dr. Williams explains the mechanism briefly and clearly: "Lecithin (phospholipids) has been proven by many studies to play a major role in maintaining the stability and clarity of the blood system. Phospholipids are found in every tissue of the body and are an important constituent of all tissue cells, including those of the brain and nerves. Because of its emulsifying capacity, lecithin acts to reduce the size of the lipid particles in the bloodstream, thus acting to inhibit or improve the atherosclerotic condition."

PATIENTS RECOVER WITH LECITHIN

Large amounts of lecithin were given to high-cholesterol patients as well as those with normal amounts in their bloodstream as part of a control group by L. A. Simons, M.D. and associates at the University of New South Wales Medical School and St. Vincent's Hospital Lipid Clinic in Sydney, Australia. (All lecithin was taken from a soybean source which also offered high amounts of unsaturated oils.)

Dr. Simons said that those with elevated blood cholesterol showed dramatic improvement. His program specified three-quarters of an ounce of lecithin granules daily. In many of the patients and the normal individuals, there was a significant drop in cholesterol levels—as much as 18 percent.

Most exciting, said Dr. Simons, was that lecithin helped reduce the so-called low-density lipoproteins or LDLs which are believed responsible for artery disease and heart trouble. This was encouraging and lecithin could well be called a heart and life saver. (*Australia and New Zealand Journal of Medicine*, June 1977.)

Why does lecithin work?

Reasons cited include (1) It has the ability to keep fat-like particles in clear solution while they journey through the arteries. In this suspension, the cholesterol-particles are unable to settle out and form dangerous deposits of fatty plaque on the walls of the blood vessels. (2) Lecithin also contains linoleic acid, a substance that is able to reduce cholesterol levels and make the blood less "sticky" and thereby lessen the risk of clots. (3) Lecithin forms a biological watchdog or "ester" inside the body that is able to metabolize already-formed fatty deposits on artery walls and carry them away.

DOCTORS, SCIENTISTS PRAISE LECITHIN

- Researchers from the UCLA Schools of Medicine and Public Health in Los Angeles tell us, "The data demonstrate that long-term ingestion of large amounts of soybean lecithin is well tolerated. This diet has been associated with lowering of serum cholesterol and triglyceride levels and a return of lipoprotein electrophoreses (measurement of protein) to normal in the patients studied." Patients consumed 48 grams of lecithin daily and showed desirable changes in their blood chemistry. (*Clinical Research*, Vol 21, p. 276.)

- Lecithin (more than corn oil) was able to reduce the risk of atherosclerosis both by lowering the LDLs and then raising the HDLs in the test women. The team of researchers found corn oil had no affect on the harmful HDLs, according to Marian T. Childs, Ph.D. with the University of Washington (Seattle) Northwest Lipid Research Clinic. (*Clinical Research*, Vol. 25, p. 159A.)

- Patients who had elevated cholesterol levels and took lecithin showed a significant drop in the blood cholesterol levels although they continued to eat a high-fat diet, reports Francis M. Pottenger, M.D. This does NOT mean you can eat foods with high fat content and take lecithin and remain immune from cholesterol overload. But it does show that lecithin can help control accumulations. (*American Journal of Digestive Diseases*, April, 1952, pp. 107-109.)

- Lecithin was able to bring about an appreciable drop in blood fats in a number of patients. Twenty-one patients with very high blood fat levels were given lecithin supplements covering a span of 120 days.

Results: Eleven out of seventeen patients with high cholesterol and eight out of twelve with high triglycerides had levels returned to normal, thanks to lecithin. (*Current Therapeutic Research*, August 1978.)

A PERSONAL EXPERIENCE WITH LECITHIN

In *Lecithin and Health*, Edward R. Hewitt has this to say about his observation of this wonder food:

"I have observed several cases where mental ills were greatly improved or entirely cured by sufficient lecithin in the diet. I myself have observed that my memory is better than it was before I took lecithin regularly. My nervous reactions are still perfectly normal at age eighty-eight. My hands are much steadier than those of any doctor who has tested me.

Blood Pressure, Arteries. "My blood pressure is from 125 to 130 over 80, and my doctor finds that my arteries show no signs of hardening and are as elastic as those of a person of forty. He also finds that he can feel the pulse in my ankles as well as in the wrist. He tells me that this is entirely unusual in a person over eighty.

"He has measured the elasticity of the arteries with a special instrument and found that they are still as elastic as those of a young man. I certainly attribute these conditions to my taking of lecithin for so long a time. My five brothers and sisters who all died around the age of seventy all had more or less circulatory difficulties. None of them lived on any regular diet.

"When ample lecithin is supplied in the diet over a long time, I have observed in many cases that the hardening in the arteries is greatly decreased and high blood pressures become much lower, in many cases returning to normal in a few months or a year or so.

"I have seen dozens of high blood pressure cases entirely cured by the use of lecithin. It must not be supposed that lecithin is a universal cure for high blood pressure. There is another type of HBP which is due to an imbalance of the two hormones secreted by the cortex of the kidney which, in a normal person, maintain the proper blood pressure. If a person has this type of HBP, lecithin is not likely to effect a cure. However, according to my own observation, more than half the HBP cases seem to be due to cholesterol, and if they are, they seem to be cured by lecithin in the diet if taken in the right amounts and for a long enough time."

Lecithin promotes healing. Edward R. Hewitt also tells of the case of his cousin who had a dangerously high blood pressure of 285 over 135. He suffered severe nose bleeds and had to spend a month in the hospital to try to get them under control. His doctors sent him home with no hope of improvement.

"I persuaded him to take one teaspoon of lecithin daily. It is good food and can do no harm. He did not receive any other treatment. In another three months, he was so much better that he could return to his office work. In a year and a half, his blood pressure had returned to 160 over 100 which is fairly good for a person fifty-nine years of age. He is still perfectly well, and looks better than he ever has since I have known him."

Hewitt says, "The time of the cure seems to be very variable. With some people, great improvement is observed in only a few weeks. With others, it is six months or more before any real improvement takes place." But we do know that improvement does occur, sooner or later. And frequently it is sooner.

Yes, lecithin may well be the miracle food of this era. Use it to cleanse your arteries and to breathe new life into your aging cells.

4 The "Dr. Rinse Lecithin Breakfast" for a Longer Life

IN 1951, a noted chemist, Dr. Jacobus Rinse, experienced his first attack of angina pectoris (chest pain) while taking a walk one windswept and chilly November day. At fifty-one, Dr. Rinse with a friend went for their "constitutional." They made their way uphill against the wind. For a while, it was smooth going. Then, Dr. Rinse felt the stabbing chest pain. More pains occurred. He had to stop and catch his breath. In a few moments he resumed the walk with his friend.

But soon he felt more sharp and penetrating pains around his heart. Dr. Jacobus Rinse was forced to sit down on the curb. He felt like fainting. His friend hailed a passing motorist who brought him home. The next few days, he experienced more and more pains. These were diagnosed by his physician as "angina pectoris." The instructions were to take prescribed medication and return in another month.

Dr. Rinse obeyed his doctor's orders. A month later, he underwent various stress exercises. "Step up, step down," directed the doctor. Dr. Rinse experienced a sharp pain. The cardiologist announced, "Now I see it." But Dr. Rinse lamented, "Now I *feel* it!" The doctor diagnosed angina pectoris and prescribed *dicumarol* (anti-coagulants to keep blood from clotting) and nitro-glycerol tablets (to keep the heart pumping).

Given when a blood vessel is plugged up by a clot, an anti-coagulant tends to prevent new clots from forming, or the existing clots from enlarging, but does NOT dissolve an existing clot. Nitroglycerin is a drug which relaxes the muscles in the blood vessels: it is a vasodila-tor. It is used to relieve attacks of angina pectoris and spasm of coronary arteries.

The doctor then pronounced the sentence: "Avoid all physical exertion, take these medications, and you should have about ten more years left to live." It was a tragic pronouncement, to say the least.

Searching for a natural way to promote heart health

Dr. Rinse refused this sentence. He decided to search for a way to overcome his distress. He knew how to conduct research; born in Amsterdam, Netherlands, he had attended the University of Amsterdam where he studied chemistry and physics. After spending a year at Johns Hopkins University and at the Bureau of Tests and the International Paper Company, he returned to Holland as chief chemist of a paint factory. In 1938, he established himself as an independent consulting chem-ist with W. Dorst in Haarlem, Netherlands. After the war, he emigrated to the U.S.A., and founded, with three other Dutch associates, a consulting laboratory in New Jersey. He directed a chemical research program until 1972 and then moved to Vermont. But let us go back to 1951 when he was given only ten years to live, even with chemotherapy.

The doctor's discoveries. Dr. Rinse did research to learn that it was cholesterol deposits that hindered circulation. (In 1951 such research was scarcely made available or known.) He learned that anginal pain is comparable to a form of heart failure in which the heart does not receive adequate oxygen for the work it is asked to do. Narrowing or contraction of the small heart arteries (arterioles) leads to chest pain or pressure.

Angina pectoris is an episode of chest pain due to a temporary discrepancy between the supply and demand of oxygen to the heart. This may be due to low oxygen levels in the blood (from smoking or respiratory disease), to a restricted bloodflow to the heart (coronary insufficiency) or to an increase in heart work beyond normal levels. Most often, angina pectoris is a chronic condition caused by restriction of the blood supply by hardening and narrowing of the coronary arteries supplying the heart muscle (coronary atherosclerosis).

The patient is dissatisfied. Dr. Rinse realized that causes of angina pectoris could be traced to too much physical activity, emotional excitement, cold weather, smoking, being overweight and a having family history of the disease. But he did not see the relevance of these causes to his case. "None of them applied to me because I kept myself calm, avoided cold weather, did not smoke, had normal weight and no family history of the ailment."

Dr. Rinse took the small pellet of nitroglycerin which he placed beneath his tongue for speedy absorption. It was carried to his heart's arterioles which were soon dilated. "The pain disappeared but sometimes the treatment needed to be repeated in fifteen to thirty minutes. I was not satisfied to make use of these small pellets the rest of my life—only ten years."

Dr. Rinse learned that his problem could be traced to *cholesterol* and its blockage of the heart and lung arteries. This latter was a problem since lung arteries transport blood needed for fuel and oxygen by the heart so it can continue pumping required blood throughout the body.

Dr. Rinse reasoned that if diet and body chemistry could cause such fat buildups, then a changed body chemistry could also reverse it. He set about in search of natural ways to help protect against cholesterol accumulation.

Supplements are helpful

Raw food diet. He decided to try raw foods (good sources of fat-melting enzymes) and subsisted on various uncooked fruits, vegetables and also took raw herring, raw meat, raw eggs, yogurt and other items. (These last named raw animal foods are not advisable under any circumstances since they contain parasites which should be killed by cooking.) Dr. Rinse found some help in raw foods. He took one supplement—*garlic*—and found that it helped him increase his span of physical activity before experiencing any anginal pain.

Vitamin C. Dr. Rinse started to take 1000 milligrams of ascorbic acid (vitamin C) daily.

Multivitamin. He then began to take a multivitamin every single day with good benefits.

Vitamin E. Having heard of the work of Evan Shute, M.D. and Wilfred E. Shute, M.D., of London, Ontario, Canada who healed countless patients of heart trouble with vitamin E, he began an exchange of correspondence. The doctors recommended that Dr. Jacobus Rinse take 200 milligrams of vitamin E after each meal.

The recovery was incomplete

For several years, Dr. Rinse took supplements—

garlic, vitamin C, multivitamin, vitamin E—and now says, "By avoiding overly strenuous exercise, I managed to live a more or less normal life. It's true that an occasional anginal warning would let me know that more heart failure was always a possibility. But I kept tabs on myself by using my pulse rate as a control. If it measured over 110, I took a rest because a rate of 65 was my normal. I took a rest also if I noticed any pressure within my chest." He thought that the use of supplements and better self-care would ease his problem. It did . . . for a while.

Early in 1957, he was struck with a heavy pain in his heart. It eased after an hour. But there were frequent recurrences of his angina pain, particularly when he climbed stairs. He experienced heart spasms and an increase of 50 strokes in his pulse rate. The pain was often so excruciating that he had to sit down and rest after completing some physical effort. He was slow to recover. So it was, that Dr. Jacobus Rinse set about to solve his continuing problem. Out of a near-fatal set of circumstances came the discovery of a miracle heart- and life-saver.

THE HEALING POWER OF LECITHIN

Dr. Rinse learned that tests had been conducted upon animals with induced heart-cholesterol difficulties. A soybean-derived substance, *lecithin*, had been administered with the report that the cholesterol could be dissolved and that health could be improved. Dr. Rinse started to do more research on *lecithin* and its reported healing powers. He started to take lecithin himself.

He took just one tablespoon of lecithin every single day, along with his other supplements. He also took one tablespoon of safflower oil which researchers said contained beneficial polyunsaturated fatty acids, required for liquefying cholesterol deposits. "Excellent results began to appear within a few days," reports Dr. Rinse.

Lecithin made the difference

Furthermore, Dr. Rinse says, "My angina pains ceased. My galloping pulse rate decreased only slightly but noticeably." He continued on his food supplement program with the addition of lecithin and safflower oil and enjoyed recuperative improvements. Three months later, his angina pectoris symptoms disappeared—even exercising failed to bring their recurrence. He traced his recovery to the use of lecithin which had turned the tide.

This supplement program was considered a success. A year later, he could even do heavy outdoor work and running. He proudly declares, "I have had no recurrence of angina or other diseases. It seems that the atherosclerotic plaques which had been narrowing my arteries to cause heart failure have been reversed."

"I am convinced that the food supplement developed in my own kitchen is a preventive and cure for atherosclerosis. It could be mixed in your kitchen, too."

Why does lecithin and supplemental program work?

According to Dr. Rinse, the amount of lecithin in the blood has much to do with the solubility of cholesterol. By daily intake of his supplemental program, the consistency of cholesterol was kept at a liquid at body temperature so that it did not get deposited on the walls of the blood vessels. Further existing atherosclerosis is then reversed.

It is *lecithin* that creates this dynamic action within the bloodstream and body.

DR. JACOBUS RINSE TELLS US . . .

Reporting his experiences to the *American Laboratory* (July 1973), and in his publication *Dietary Counterattack Against Atherosclerosis*, Dr. Rinse offers these comments on the success of his lecithin supplemental program:

"The human body is comparable to a chemical plant, producing various kinds of energies for moving and thinking, for electric energy, and for heat . . .

"The human body needs secondary materials such as minerals, metals, vitamins and enzymes. These are needed to run the numerous chemical reactions of metabolism, for the production of energy, and in particular for the digestion of proteins, fats and carbohydrates, which are the primary raw materials for the body. Therefore, food must contain everything in adequate quantities and should be varied as much as possible."

What about cholesterol?

Being chemically minded, this respected physicist has this view: "Although statistically the chance for atherosclerosis (hardening of the arteries) is higher if the cholesterol content of blood is high, many persons are healthy with a high cholesterol count.

"Therefore, it is doubtful whether the efforts to lower cholesterol content by all means are justified. Such efforts include avoidance of food containing cholesterol— such as eggs and butter, or using drugs that effect the production of cholesterol in the liver.

"It has been demonstrated that the liver produces more cholesterol if food contains less. Reducing its production by the liver by means of drugs can be dangerous and has caused serious side effects like cataracts and hair loss. It seems that you cannot change cholesterol production in your body without penalty.

The lecithin cholesterol compound. "On the other hand, if lecithin is added to the diet, the unwanted deposits of cholesterol derivatives do not form, because the lecithin-cholesterol compound is soluble. Both materials occur in eggs. Therefore, an atherosclerotic patient should not deprive himself of eating eggs. We have seen that polyunsaturated oil should be present. Any excess of cholesterol in the bloodstream is removed from the body through the intestines."

Dr. Rinse adds with emphasis: *"Only in the presence of sufficient lecithin can polyunsaturated fatty acid help in dissolving cholesterol."*

THE FAMOUS DR. RINSE BREAKFAST

Dr. Rinse prepared his own breakfast which he feels has saved him from impending fatalities. He says that this combination of vitamins and minerals can be "beneficial for the cure and prevention of atherosclerotic complications such as high blood pressure, angina pectoris, cataracts and obstructions in the arteries of the neck, legs, arms and kidneys. The end result can be the reduction or avoidance of heart trouble and cerebral thrombosis."

Here is how you can mix it, based on Dr. Rinse's complete recipe.

Basic Mixture: Combine one part each of: soybean lecithin, debittered brewer's yeast, raw wheat germ, bone meal. Mix together and refrigerate in a closed container. Prepare only a small amount at a time.

Your breakfast:

> In a bowl, mix:
> 2 tablespoons of Basic Mixture
> 1 tablespoon dark-brown sugar (this might be eliminated; use a bit of honey as a substitute, if desired)
> 1 tablespoon of safflower oil or any other linoleate oil (soybean oil, for example)
> Enough milk to dissolve sugar and yeast
> Enough yogurt to increase consistency
> Add cold cereal for calories, as needed, or mix with hot cereal such as porridge or oatmeal. Add sun-dried raisins or fruit as desired
> (For severe atherosclerosis, double amount of lecithin.)

Suggestion: Have this nutrient-packed, lecithin-powerful Dr. Rinse breakfast every single day. It will do much to help keep your arteries clean and your heart healthfully alive.

Dr. Rinse says, "Any other normal food may be used" in your daily diet, "including eggs and butter, but high-melting fats such as regular margarine and deep-frying fats must be avoided. Soft margarines such as those containing linoleate (read labels) are helpful. Butter is preferred because it contains medium-chain-triglycerides (MCT) fat."

Supplements to take daily

> 500 milligrams vitamin C
> 100 units vitamin E
> 1 multivitamin-mineral tablet

Answer your own needs

"Each person must decide, from his own experimentation, what mixture of ingredients should be part of the daily intake. An individual's metabolism may require extra quantities of minerals or more vitamins. For example, during the winter, some people feel they need more vitamin C to offset influenza dangers. If a nervous disorder is present, a person might add a high concentration of vitamin B-complex to the suggested mixture."

When to take breakfast? Not necessarily at breakfast, if your taste buds crave another delight. Dr. Rinse says that his formula "could be incorporated into fruit juices or in soup. Other foodstuffs can be added to it to enhance flavor. Dried or fresh fruits might be eaten with it. The mixture might be made a part of Swiss-type cereals like Muesli. These Muesli preparations are excellent since they are likely to contain most of the required vitamins and minerals, although not always in the proper quantities."

Enjoy foods but not to excess. It is this learned chemist's feeling that most any food can be eaten, unless special conditions require their avoidance. Generally speaking, he said, you need not limit intake of butter, eggs, milk, cream, but "take precaution against excesses of these foods." He advises sufficient amounts of protein, fats and carbohydrates.

Why do his recommendations work?

Dr. Rinse's selection of supplements are aimed at creating a dietary counterattack against atherosclerosis. They prevent the accumulation of cholesterol. These supplements, says Dr. Rinse, bring about a dissolution of the cholesterol plaques.

In particular, lecithin and linoleate oils (such as safflower) create that action. They are synergistic (combine their action) with all other ingredients in the mixture. Each component strengthens or fortifies the other.

"No other changes in the diet are needed when the food supplements are used," says Dr. Rinse.

He then tells us, "Atherosclerosis is a deficiency disease which can be counteracted successfully by the use of food supplements, in particular lecithin and unsaturated fats."

LECITHIN + OIL MELT CHOLESTEROL

In the Rinse Breakfast, you'll notice the need for a combination of both lecithin and oil. Why is this so important?

Cholesterol and lecithin need to combine in the presence of adequate amounts of linoleate (safflower or other oils). When they do, there is a melting point below body temperature.

Caution: Without the availability of the oil, cholesterol has a very high melting point and may form insoluble plaques in arterial walls.

Whether in or outside the arterial walls, lecithin plus oils are needed to help melt away cholesterol. That is, the dissolving of cholesterol is possible with the oil-lecithin presence. In the presence of oil, the melting point for cholesterol drops to 0°C. or 32°F. This is far below body temperature and thus facilitates the melting of this fat. Without oil, cholesterol is not that easy to melt. Therefore, you need this combination—lecithin plus oil. This is the foundation of the Rinse Breakfast.

THE DOCTOR'S RECOMMENDATIONS

As living proof of the heart-saving powers of lecithin, Dr. Rinse now gives us his summarized recommendations for a longer and healthier lifeline:

1. Atherosclerosis is a deficiency disease which can be prevented or reversed by the ingestion of lecithin and polyunsaturated (linoleate) oils. These tend to dissolve cholesterol deposits in the arteries.

2. Lecithin and polyunsaturated oil should be used in conjunction with antioxidant food supplements such as vitamins C and E.

3. Modern food, since it is overprocessed and deficient in essential food elements as a result, should be supplemented with all of the known vitamins and minerals.

4. A combination of fortified nutrients which may be designated as the anti-atherosclerotic food formula has favorable influence on altering the atherosclerotic process.

5. By combining the formula ingredients—yeast, wheat germ, bone meal, lecithin, linoleate oil, raw sugar (optional), milk, yogurt, vitamins C and E, and multivitamins—a synergistic effect is obtained. This will permit a more therapeutic reaction from smaller quantities of each component than if they were taken separately. (Again, emphasis is on the *combination* of these nutrients rather than just taking them individually.)

6. Atherosclerosis is reversible in the less advanced cases where the arteries have not lost their flexibility. A full range of activities might be resumed with consump-

tion of the anti-atherosclerotic food formula as a daily routine.

7. Within certain limits, no restrictions hold for any kind of food, even butter, milk, cream and eggs. This is the rule if the recommended food supplements are ingested routinely.

(NOTE: You are advised to consult with your family physician regarding your individual diet regimen for your particular health condition.)

Dr. Jacobus Rinse was given ten years to live in 1951. He is today three decades later more alive, more vigorous, more energetic than ever before. It is the Rinse Breakfast and especially the use of lecithin that has helped him live longer—and better!

5

How You Can Enjoy Vim-Vigor-Vitality with Lecithin

DO YOU WANT to wake up in the morning with a feeling of youthful vitality? Do you want to have alert emotional health? Do you want to have "staying power" of both body and mind for as long as is healthfully possible? There is a way that this can be yours with the use of lecithin. When you understand that this substance is found in every living cell, then you realize how essential it is that lecithin be provided for every part of your body. When you are "nourished" with lecithin, you enjoy vitality—at any age.

Prevalence of lecithin. The highest concentrations are found in the organs that perform the most essential functions of daily living. For example, your brain, if dried and analyzed, would show a composition of about 30 percent lecithin. High concentrations are also found in your heart, liver, kidneys, nerves and muscles. When you "lecithin-ize" these organs, you then invigorate your entire body.

Lecithin in your diet

Although there is little doubt that lecithin *must* be present in your body to perform a vital role in fat and nutritive metabolism, a natural and balanced diet should provide the raw materials necessary for your body to synthesize its own.

Good sources. Unprocessed seeds, nuts and whole grains, unrefined seed oils, organ meats and other fat-containing animal products are all good sources of lecithin. But animal fats, like those of meat, eggs and butter also contain cholesterol. By trying to avoid high-cholesterol foods, you may actually be limiting the amounts of lecithin obtained from the diet. Even worse, the lecithin naturally present in many foods is often removed or destroyed during commercial processing.

You want to enjoy metabolic-induced vim and vigor. You need lecithin. Granules are suggested to help make up for the deficiency.

THE "VIM INGREDIENT" IN LECITHIN

Soybean lecithin contains a combination of soy phosphatides, including phosphatidyl choline, phosphatidyl inositol and others. The one "vim ingredient" is that of *phosphatidyl choline*, the most powerful element in this wonder food.

In 1975, researchers at Massachusetts Institute of Technology made an unexpected discovery. The amounts of choline in the body can influence vitality of the brain and general body behavior. How is this possible?

Choline and your brain

Putting it simply, choline is required by your brain for the production of acetylcholine, a vital compound synthesized by your brain for the transmission of messages from one nerve cell to another.

The amount of choline available to your brain depends primarily upon the amount of lecithin recently eaten. Apparently, if more acetylcholine is available for the transmission of a nerve message, more information can be carried in each impulse.

This is the reason why some folks are more energetic in body and mind than others. They have more lecithin-created acetylcholine which is used to energize the brain and body.

This same lecithin-created acetylcholine is believed to be involved in a wide range of normal brain activities including learning, memory, sensory feedback, motor coordination, sleep and arousal, hormonal secretions and the regulation of various body functions such as respiration, circulation and digestion.

Brain biochemists are finding increasing evidence that a variety of brain and bodily disorders may result from the inability of the brain to produce or utilize sufficient acetylcholine.

The impact of these discoveries was summarized by one MIT researcher when he commented at a symposium on Dietary Choline Sources and Brain Function held at MIT in November 1977: "It comes as a surprise that Nature would allow our dietary habits to control such a vital function as neurotransmitter synthesis."

In other words, the more acetylcholine you have, the more alert and active is your brain and also your body.

CHOLINE DEFICIENCY LEADS TO LIVER MALFUNCTION

"It is known from histological and biochemical evidence that withdrawal of choline from the diet in one single meal causes accumulation of lipid (fat) in the liver," says Dr. Sailen Mookerjea of the Medical Research Department of the Charles H. Best Institute of the University of Toronto. As reported in *Federation*

Proceedings (January-February 1971), the doctor says that tests show that "the increase of liver lipids within one or two days of choline deprivation, uncomplicated by unnecessary manipulations, has always been an irreproachable fact."

When your liver becomes choline-deficient, your entire body health starts to decline. This explains why lecithin-nourished folks are energetic (because of choline intake) and others are always tired (because of choline deficiency and liver malfunction).

As explained before, choline is a basic substance in lecithin, the wonder food that your body cannot do without. With lecithin-supplied choline, you can then enjoy a healthy liver and youthful metabolic process.

WHAT LECITHIN CHOLINE MEANS TO YOUR HEALTH

When you are nourished with lecithin, its supply of choline can make all the difference between youthful vitality and senile tiredness. That is precisely how essential choline can be for your body.

According to the noted chemist Dr. C. W. Whitmoyer, Fellow of the American Institute of Chemists and author of *Your Health Is What You Make It:*

"Choline is biologically important for several reasons. It serves as the precursor of acetylcholine, which performs an important function in the transmission of nerve impulses across neuromuscular junctions.

"Choline serves as a source of methyl (chemical) groups for the synthesis of several important biological substances, probably in the synthesis of the hormone apinephrine (adrenalin), and particularly in the synthesis of the essential amino acid methionine.

"Choline is a component of phospholipids which are essential substances for the transport of fatty acids in the blood so that they may be deposited at the proper site, especially to the liver, adipose tissue and nerve tissue."

Dr. Whitmoyer adds that one typical phospholipid is that of lecithin. He says that in its absence there is the accumulation of excess neutral fat and cholesterol in the liver.

Therefore, we see that choline influences your nerve impulses (the very act of moving your eyes across this page, the desire to turn the page are some of the millions of motions influenced by choline) and also is involved in liver fat metabolism. You do need choline. You do need lecithin which is a prime source of this energy-boosting nutrient.

NATURAL VS. SYNTHETIC CHOLINE

Yes, there is a difference! To know why natural is preferred, read on.

Basic facts

Choline can be produced synthetically in the form of compounds containing relatively large percentages of pure choline. Examples of these are choline chloride, choline bitartrate, and choline dihydrogen citrate.

Over 99 percent of the choline naturally obtained in the diet is in the form of soybean lecithin—more precisely, *phosphatidyl choline*.

Lecithin attaches to a specific compound of definite structure—phosphatidyl choline. The phosphatide mixture of commercial lecithin contains about 29 percent of phosphatidyl choline—actual lecithin—in the oil-free form, and only about 18 percent actual lecithin in the liquid form with a carrier of soybean oil. For a power-house of choline, it is important to use lecithin granules.

After discovering the relationship of dietary choline to brain function, the MIT researchers tested the effectiveness of different forms of choline in raising and maintaining blood choline levels.

Case history sited

As reported in *Lancet* (July 9, 1977), young, healthy volunteers at MIT ingested equal amounts of choline either as choline chloride (one of the synthetic choline compounds) or lecithin granules (pure form) and fasted for the next twelve hours.

"In the subjects who took choline chloride (synthetic), serum choline levels reached its peak (86 percent above normal levels) after thirty minutes, but was not significantly higher than normal after four hours.

"In those who took lecithin (pure form), the first significant rise in serum choline levels occurred after one hour, but peak levels (265 percent above normal) persisted for at least twelve hours."

These scientists tell us, "We report here that the consumption of lecithin (pure), the major dietary source of choline, is much more effective than choline chloride (synthetic) in raising serum choline levels."

There is a difference

In the prestigious journal *Science* (October 13, 1978), a team of researchers pointed out that there is a difference between natural and synthetic:

"The metabolic fate of choline consumed as (natural) lecithin apparently differs from that of free (synthetic) choline. A major fraction of orally ingested choline is rapidly degraded in the human intestine by a bacterial enzyme to yield trimethylamine, a compound with a marked fishy odor; in contrast, the consumption of choline as (pure) lecithin does not give subjects a fishy odor and causes much greater increase in plasma choline per molecule consumed, than does choline chloride."

Therefore, pure lecithin is more effective than synthetic choline.

GETTING TO KNOW TRUE LECITHIN

To boost body energy, you should use true or pure lecithin, the best source of vitality.

Remember, just about all choline obtained in the diet is consumed in the form of *phosphatidyl choline*. This is found in lecithin granules. Scientists already recognize that only one phosphatide is true lecithin—that of phosphatidyl choline.

It should be emphasized that phosphatidyl choline is the only component of lecithin of value to brain biochemists and cardiovascular researchers. It is true that all lecithin products contain a mixture of phosphatides. But only *one* is regarded as true lecithin: phosphatidyl choline.

When selecting your product, read the label. If it contains natural soybean phosphatides and natural phosphatidyl choline, then it is the same high-potency, vigor-producing lecithin that is lauded by researchers and scientists. It is the product you will want to improve your capacities.

Forms of lecithin re-examined

Liquid or capsules do not provide natural choline

(source of energy of body and mind) in as concentrated a form as pure lecithin granules.

Granules are 50 percent more concentrated and contain 43 percent fewer calories than liquid lecithin.

Ten 1200 milligram capsules are required to equal the potency of a single tablespoon (7.5 grams) of granules.

The "high potency soya lecithin granules" usually consist of defatted soy flour and offer you 400 milligrams of choline per tablespoon—by the addition of synthetic choline!

So it would appear that for good terms of nutritional value, potency, convenience and palatability, the pure lecithin granules should be favored. Legally speaking, pure lecithin granules must contain at least 90 percent soy phosphatides. So you're assured of high-potency phosphatidyl choline (read labels!) when buying the pure lecithin granules.

LECITHIN AND METABOLISM

You may eat a balanced diet and still feel tired. The reason here is that you have poor or weak metabolism. The nutrients in foods cannot be properly absorbed by your bloodstream to provide you with important energy. You need the power of lecithin. The lecithin present in the body plays a dynamic part in the metabolism and transport of fatty substances. How can this work?

You know that water and oil do not readily mix. Your body consists of about 70 percent water, yet fats and oils are essential. How can the fats function in this environment? The answer lies first in the remarkable emulsifying properties of lecithin, whereby one end of the molecule (containing fatty acids) is attracted to the oil and the other end (containing phosphorus and nitrogen) is attracted to the water; and second in the associations of lecithin with protein. Dietary lecithin provides essential building blocks as well as aiding in the absorption of fats and fat-soluble vitamins.

Indeed, there is a relationship in fat metabolism between choline, inositol, phosphorus compounds and fatty acids. When present together in your diet, each of these four factors has a better effect than they do in isolation. Lecithin granules provide all of these factors. Lecithin thus acts as a sort of "bridge" between water and oil, and this makes it a pathway to the enjoyment of youthful vim and vigor.

6

How to "Think Young" and Protect against Senility with Lecithin

○━━━━━○━○━━━━━○━○━━━━━○

DOES YOUR MEMORY seem fuzzy at times? Do you have difficulties in remembering faces, facts, dates, numbers? Do you experience memory lapses when your mind is just a blank? The cause could be traced to a nutritional deficiency. Your brain, like the rest of your body organs, requires a specific set of nutrients in order to function with youthful vitality. In particular, there are nutrients in lecithin that appear to help you "think young" and protect you against so-called senility. To better understand how lecithin's nutrients are so brain-nourishing, you need to know a few basic facts about this "think tank," the second most important organ (after your heart) in your body.

GETTING TO KNOW YOUR BRAIN

Its name is derived from a combination of Old English and Greek words *bregen* and *brechmos*, meaning the "front part of the head."

Basically, your brain is the portion of your central nervous system that constitutes the organ of thought and neural coordination.

Your body computer. Your brain is more than just a

63

source of your thoughts. It is your body computer. It consists of over 12 *billion* cells which function as batteries, resistors, transformers and switchers. (The average TV set has less than twenty-five resistors and transformers so you can readily appreciate the awesome power of that compact mass of matter in your head.) Your brain weighs slightly more than three pounds and is considered a weighty power in your life.

Your brain is the controlling organ of your body. It allows you to think, reason, plan, feel, in ways that make you different from so-called lower animals. As the foundation of your mind, your brain is able to perceive, remember, combine and create at both conscious and unconscious levels. Your brain is able to direct such activities as the life-providing efficiency of your heart beat, your normal rate of breathing, your pulse rate and just about every function imaginable. (Even imagination is determined by your brain!)

Basic parts of your brain

There are basic division of your brain:

Cerebrum. Also called the forebrain, it is considered the "brain proper" and is the largest part of this organ. It fills most of the upper regions of your skull. It is divided into two segments. The *outer* shell (cerebral cortex) is about an eighth of an inch thick and consists of a solid mass of gray matter. Your cerebral cortex is the source of very high intellectual functions. The *inner* segment contains the thalamus and the hypothalamus. These act as main relay stations for sensory impulses directed to the cerebral cortex and also regulate your body's basic requirements such as temperature, sleep, water balance, digestion and assimilation of ingested foods.

Cerebellum This hindbrain is found in the lower rear position of your skull. It is needed to regulate body equilibrium and help you coordinate muscular movements. Any injury or a nutritional deficiency may cause staggering gait, trembling muscles (as in palsy) and slurred speech.

Brain stem This includes the medulla oblongata. It is the extension and upper terminal of your spinal cord and is found at your skull's base. This segment serves as a site of communication between your brain and spinal cord. It determines your life-producing functions such as breathing, heartbeat and the swallowing of food and liquids.

Within your brain stem, there is a complete set of important nerves. For example, in your brain stem, nerves originate *in* or come *from* the left side of your body and then switch over to the right side of your brain—or vice versa. Nourishment is important in order to maintain this switchover of your nerves. Otherwise, there may result a slowdown of this power and you may develop paralysis-like reactions on one side of your body.

NUTRIENTS FOR YOUTHFUL BRAIN POWER

Scientific researchers have perceived that when certain substances in your brain (the *neurotransmitters*) are deficient, nervous disorders can occur. These disorders can be directly connected to the deficiency of that particular neurostransmitter.

These researchers have found that when they give the patient substances from which the neurotransmitter is made, there is either a modification, easing or even total correction of the symptoms caused by this neurotransmitter deficiency.

For example, many emotional (physical and/or mental) disorders can be traced to a deficiency of the neurotransmitter acetylcholine, a nutrient that is largely composed from the B-complex vitamin, choline.

Scientists use lecithin. Researchers have found that when you eat lecithin for a primary and highly concentrated source of choline, there follows a metabolic reaction which causes a substantially higher level of choline in your bloodstream than if you would take a choline supplement alone. Additional studies show that the lecithin choline creates higher levels of much needed acetylcholine in your brain. This may well be the key to helping you "think young" and protecting yourself against so-called "senility."

Case study reported. A team of psychiatrists treated patients suffering from tardive dyskinesia, an impairment of voluntary movement caused by the use of a psychiatric drug. The doctors say that lecithin was able to cause easing of symptoms, much more effectively than choline by itself. Also, the doctors note that large doses of choline may cause digestive upset. But the use of lecithin caused no symptoms, except some weight gain in one patient. That TD was eased with the use of choline-rich lecithin was important news. (*American Journal of Psychiatry*, June 1979.)

LECITHIN HELPS CORRECT SENILITY

The use of lecithin was able to offer appreciably beneficial correction of so-called senility (impaired learning ability) in three out of seven patients diagnosed as having "presenile dementia." In this problem, there is a slow deterioration of the brain. Mental capacities wane. If unchecked, the person may even suffer from hallucinations.

The doctors administered lecithin with its high supply of choline and reported, "During the tests, they seemed to understand instructions faster and more clearly, their verbal rambling was less striking and they were more cooperative." (*Lancet*, December 2, 1978)

Why did this produce such beneficial results? The lecithin choline appeared to send a supply of much needed acetylcholine to nourish the neurotransmitters of the brain. Once amply invigorated, neurotransmitters may now receive and send messages with youthful gusto. This may be the clue to correction of so-called memory problems. Furthermore, lecithin is able to promote a more healthful flow of blood through the arteries and protects against congestion which can also interfere with brain (and body) health.

SCIENTISTS USE LECITHIN FOR BRAIN POWER

Not only can choline help treat problems of what could be disabling brain disorders, but it can also "nourish" the brain to ease problems such as emotional depression and memory defects.

As reported in the New York *Times* (January 26, 1978), scientists have found that choline is able to pass into your bloodstream from food in your digestive tract. But something interesting occurs in your metabolic process. The choline is now taken directly by your brain from your circulating blood. It is biologically used to help your brain create a vital chemical transmitter of *nerve signals*. This is an around-the-clock process whereby *the youthful effectiveness of your nerve signal transmitter in your brain is influenced by the amount of choline available in your system!*

For example, you have just finished a plate of scrambled eggs (or eggs in any other form) which gives your body a high amount of choline. Within a few hours, your metabolism will have a much-needed quantity of the nerve signal transmitter called acetylcholine in your brain.

In other words, the choline is able to nourish your brain with acetylcholine.

This is important according to MIT researcher Richard J. Wurtman, M.D. "It means that the composition of each meal will directly affect the synthesis of chemical signals in your brain." Or—what you eat is what you think in a few hours!

Furthermore, the availability of this nutrient (choline) means "an amplification of the nerve signals sent from one nerve cell to the next by those cells that use acetylcholine for the signaling."

CASE STUDIES OF NERVOUS DISORDERS

This research is based on the treatments administered to people troubled with tardive dyskinesia (TD). As we have explained, this condition is seen in mental patients under treatment with drugs (the anti-psychotic chemicals such as the phenothiazines or the butyrophenones). Mental patients may be given either of these drugs to help calm them down and also ease their reactions to mental illness. After months or years of being under this chemotherapy, these mental patients develop uncontrollable jerking movements of the upper body and limbs. There are unusual facial gestures and bizarre tongue movements.

Since these persons are already troubled with emotional disorder, such physical jerks and spasms can make them feel much worse. But science could not find an antidote. To compound the problem, many persons became *permanently* afflicted with TD even after drugs were discontinued.

It is said that as many as 40 percent of older and terminally institutionalized mental patients under this chemotherapy developed TD. Furthermore, if these drugs are prescribed for outpatients, they, too, run the risk of developing what could be permanent *tardive dyskinesis*.

The MIT scientists explain that TD presumably is traced to a failure of brain nerve cells to release adequate amounts of acetylcholine. Therefore, Dr. Richard J. Wurtman tested animals and found that when they had "extra blood choline," there was an increase in the release of amounts of this brain transmitter substance, acetylcholine. Dr. Wurtman and a team of scientists conducted a very carefully controlled study with the use of choline. It was their hope that this nutrient would release amounts of acetylcholine and create healthy neurotransmitters.

In the study, nine TD patients were given choline for a period of about fourteen days. The doctors report that these patients "showed major improvements." Of course, some patients showed no change (one became worse) but Dr. Wurtman adds, "This indicates that in this group of patients were included conditions stemming from something more complex than the classic TD."

Dr. Wurtman and his staff felt very encouraged about these results and decided to use *lecithin* as a prime source of choline.

CHOLINE AND BRAIN HEALTH

In view of the above results, other scientists are

researching the connection between choline and brain health. Dr. David Drachman of the University of Massachusetts at Worcester feels that choline may help prevent memory loss among persons who have varying levels of so-called senility.

Choline may also influence two basic forms of mental illness: so-called manic and then depressive states. Dr. John Davis of the University of Chicago theorizes that both of these conditions result from a derangement of a balance between two important nerve signal transmitters: norepinephrine and acetylcholine. Specifically, choline levels are too high in depression and norepinephrine levels are too high in mania. There is believed to be a metabolic-digestive error that causes this uneven balance.

But these researchers do agree that acetylcholine is a decisive influence on brain health.

According to Richard J. Wurtman, M.D., and co-researcher, Madelyn J. Hirsch, in *Science* (Vol. 202, pp. 223-24), the use of lecithin will increase acetylcholine concentrations in the brain and also a adrenal gland, as performed on test animals. Consumption of just a single meal containing lecithin, the major source of choline occurring naturally in the diet, increased the concentrations of choline and acetylcholine in the brain and adrenal gland.

Dr. Wurtman says that "the consumption for three to eleven days of a diet supplemented with choline chloride increases the concentration of serum choline, brain choline and brain acetylcholine."

As for using lecithin as a source of phosphatidylcholine, it appears to be more potent. Also, it frees you from the "marked fishy odor" coming from the choline chloride.

There is reported a much greater increase in plasma choline with the use of lecithin as a source.

Are you getting enough choline? According to Dr. Wurtman, "high lecithin concentrations occur naturally in such foods as egg yolks (up to 1.75 percent choline), liver (0.6 percent choline) and soybeans (0.3 percent choline.) Reliable data apparently are lacking on the average total daily lecithin intake of adults. One estimate is that adults consume 0.5 to 0.9 grams of choline per day."

Dr. Wurtman says that your normal day-to-day variations in food choice could easily generate tenfold differences that "could influence cholinergic neurotransmission."

This means that you may not be eating eggs, liver and soybeans in adequate quantities for daily choline intake. Neither would you want to because these are high cholesterol foods; although the lecithin emulsification action could help metabolize the cholesterol, it would be impractical to expect to eat these foods daily. Therefore, lecithin is suggested as a healthy supplement.

Purity is important. Lecithin's clinical utility is enhanced if the pure compound is used. Lecithin administration might also provide a useful adjunct to existing drug therapies in disease. For example, mania, myasthenia gravis and psychosis are thought to benefit from enhanced cholinergic neurotransmission. Putting it simply, it is believed that "pure lecithin" (it contains 15 to 20 percent pure phosphatidyl choline and *is* available and at low cost), would be helpful in boosting much-needed neurotransmitters in the brain and this could help ease various ailments.

MEMORY LOSS CORRECTED BY LECITHIN

A major breakthrough in problems of memory loss was announced in the New York *Times* (January 9, 1979): the use of lecithin-choline can help correct different types of so-called senility or memory loss. A research team suggested that choline does have a decisive influence on brain health. They offered this three-step explanation:

1. *Where is choline found?* In many foods, particularly egg yolks, meat and fish.
2. *What is its special property?* Choline is able to penetrate the so-called blood-brain barrier which ordinarily protects the brain against variations in your daily food fare. In so doing, choline is able to pass directly into the cells of the brain.
3. *What is its impact on the brain?* Choline simulates specific brain cells to produce more acetylcholine, a substance that transmits nerve impulses. "There is much evidence linking cells that use acetylcholine to the formation of memory."

The amazing *power* of choline is found in its ability to *penetrate* the above-mentioned barrier and influence the brain. Few foods (alcohol is the exception, and narcotics, too) can create such a reaction.

At a 1979 three-day symposium in Tucson, Arizona on the use of choline and related substances in nerve and mental disease, these facts were presented about memory improvement:

Eases Alzheimer's disease. In this problem, there are memory problems and a mind-destroying reaction. Janice Christie, M.D., and colleagues from Edinburgh, Scotland, reported that the use of choline could help improve the memory of test subjects; at least, the progression of the illness was slowed down with choline.

Scientists of the National Institute Of Mental Health used choline on patients at St. Elizabeths Hospital of Washington, D.C., and found evidence that the memory of normal persons who had short-term memory scores could be improved.

These reports offered hope for brain and emotional health improvement with the use of choline.

NUTRITION AND BRAIN HEALTH

"Nutritional studies have made important contributions to brain science," notes John H. Growdon, M.D., assistant professor at Tufts University School of Medicine and assistant neurologist at Tufts New England Medical Center Hospital of Boston, as issued in *Nutrition Reviews*, (Vol. 37, No. 5, pp. 129-136.) "Eight years ago, we observed that the composition of each meal can influence the synthesis of the brain neurotransmitter serotonin. Subsequent studies have shown that this kind of nutritional control is fairly general."

Dr. Growdon continues to explain that nutrients from ingested food tend to stimulate this action. In particular, "choline availability in the brain directly influences the rates at which cholinergic neurons synthesize and release their neurotransmitter, acetylcholine." Therefore, choline appears to have strong influence in creating this beneficial brain-reflex reaction."

Dr. Growdon tells that "administration of choline by injection or by dietary supplementation increased blood choline, brain choline and brain acetylcholine levels in animals." He specifically points out that "choline ingested as lecithin, its naturally occurring source, was even more effective in elevating serum choline levels in humans, and brain and adrenal acetylcholine levels in animals."

The doctor tells of successful healings with the use of choline as reported by colleagues. Cited were the aforementioned tardive dyskinesia, problems of Huntington's disease, Friedreich's ataxia (an hereditary neurologic disease involving posture and movement), Alzheimer's type of dementia, to name just a few. "Lecithin is also being tested in patients with mania, since this mood disorder also shows a marked response to physostigmine medication."

Dr. John H. Growdon looks ahead when he adds, "It is likely that uses of lecithin will increase as physicians examine its effects in other diseases characterized by inadequate cholinergic neurotransmission."

This does offer hope for total healing with proper lecithin-choline intake and availability to the metabolic process.

HOW PURE IS THAT LECITHIN?

Is that lecithin really as pure as the label indicates? How can you be sure you're getting the grade and quality that will be of optimal benefit?

Here's a simple-to-read guideline offered by Dr. Growdon:

"Pure lecithin" is in reality usually only 15 to 25 percent pure phosphatidyl choline.

A quirk in labeling laws currently allows lecithin manufacturers to call any mixture containing 95 percent phosphatides "pure lecithin," even though, to the chemical and biomedical communities, the terms "lecithin" and "phosphatide" are not synonymous.

Only one phosphatide—phosphatidyl choline—directly contributes choline to your body for acetylcholine synthesis.

How can you be certain? In three words—*read the label;* If it specifies that the lecithin product is *phosphatidyl choline*, then it is the lecithin you are looking for.

Yes, you can improve your emotional health and boost the thinking powers of your brain, when you have an adequate amount of needed neurotransmitters available at all times. This is possible with the use of lecithin, the food your brain must have for total survival.

7 Questions and Answers About Lecithin

QUESTION: *In brief, what are the benefits of lecithin?*

ANSWER: The phosphatidyl choline obtained from lecithin is an important constituent of many enzymes and other essential substances produced by your body. It contributes nutrients from which, for example, acetylcholine can be produced for the transmission of nerve impulses. Lipoproteins can be formed for the transport of fat and cholesterol. Lecithin is also intimately and intricately involved in the absorption and metabolism of fats. In fact, lecithin plays a role in *every* bodily system and is present in *every* living cell.

QUESTION: *Where does lecithin come from?*

ANSWER: Lecithin, in America, is produced commercially from soybeans. It requires about 2000 pounds of soybeans to obtain five pounds of lecithin granules.

QUESTION: *How much lecithin should a person take?*

ANSWER: To begin, lecithin is found in natural, unprocessed foods so if you eat a balanced diet, you will get a reasonable amount of it. But to meet the challenges of everyday living, you may want additional amounts. Now then, the minimal daily requirement for choline has not been established, but it is estimated that the average dietary intake of this nutrient is between 400 and 900 milligrams per day. Generally speaking, two level tablespoons of lecithin granules would help assure an adequate amount of phosphatidyl choline for the average person. If you have a condition of less-than-satisfactory health, then you might want to use as much as four to six tablespoons of granules a day.

QUESTION: *Isn't there any risk of overdosage?*

ANSWER: No. Lecithin is a food and does not have side effects.

QUESTION: *What is the best way to use lecithin granules?*

ANSWER: Most people like to eat the granules right from the jar. Or mix them with any juice or beverage. The granules add very little taste of their own. They immediately lose their granular consistency and become part of the beverage within a minute or two. Lecithin granules may also be added to cereals, salads, egg dishes, mashed potatoes, yogurt or just about anything.

QUESTION: *May I add lecithin to cooked or baked foods? Will there be any loss of value?*

ANSWER: Feel free to add lecithin in all recipes. There is no value destruction during cooking or baking.

QUESTION: *Should lecithin be refrigerated?*

ANSWER: Not necessarily. Lecithin granules will remain fresh for at least a year if you follow these rules:

(1) Keep the bottle stored under 120°F. (49°C.) temperatures.

(2) Keep out of direct light.

(3) Always replace cap tightly after use.

Note: If you do refrigerate lecithin, take special care to replace the cap immediately after use to prevent moisture in the air from condensing on the granules.

QUESTION: *What is the difference between liquid lecithin, ordinary lecithin capsules and lecithin granules?*

ANSWER: Liquid lecithin is a rather inexpensive product produced for commercial use as an emulsifier in foods, cosmetics, paints, etc. It consists of approximately 61 percent phosphatides and 37 percent soybean oil. The liquid lecithin used in ordinary lecithin capsules is even lower in phosphatides since it must be diluted with even more oil to achieve the proper consistency for encapsulation.

The purest lecithin granules contain over 95 percent phosphatides and about 2 percent soybean oil. Granules are about 60 percent more concentrated and contain 45 percent fewer calories than an equal weight of liquid lecithin. Studies indicate that lecithin granules, richer in phosphatidyl choline may be more effective, and that the polyunsaturated fatty acids contained in phosphatidyl choline are better utilized in the body than those from soy or other vegetable oils.

QUESTION: *What is lecithin powder?*

ANSWER: Simply granules in powder form. This may be advantageous in some commercial applications.

CAUTION: A product labelled as "Lecithin Powder" may not be *pure* lecithin. Most such products may consist of liquid lecithin spray-dried with whey or non-fat dry milk solids, yielding a product with a low phosphatide content. If no phosphatide content is given on the label, then ask questions.

QUESTION: *Aren't there lecithin granules that contain more nutrients?*

ANSWER: Until a few years ago, all products labelled as lecithin granules contained over 95 percent soybean phosphatides. There was a time when manufacturers could not meet the demand for lecithin granules so they created a product labeled as "Lecithin Granules." This is not pure soybean phosphatides. Instead, it consists of primarily 60 to 70 percent defatted soybean flour, about 30 percent liquid lecithin and synthetic choline.

QUESTION: *Wouldn't such a product be helpful?*

ANSWER: Soy flour contains nutrients that lecithin does not, but defatted soy flour is not lecithin. Also, 400 milligrams of synthetic choline found in one table-spoon of imitation soy flour granules cannot be equal to the phosphatidyl choline provided by genuine lecithin granules.

QUESTION: *Aren't there regulations about such products?*

ANSWER: The official Food Chemical Codex requires products labelled as lecithin to contain not less than 50 percent phosphatides. These imitation granules contain only about 20 percent phosphatides. Furthermore, the FDA has issued regulatory letters ordering label changes for these products, but the orders appear not to have been complied with, or enforced. So you have to be a label reader to know the product you want and need.

QUESTION: *Aren't these weaker lecithin granules suitable or effective?*

ANSWER: Like any nutrient, you will benefit from more vigorous potencies. Such products may be fine for those who want a small amount of lecithin. But even so, most consumers are not aware of the low lecithin content; they pay for lecithin granules and receive much cheaper and less effective defatted soy flour.

QUESTION: *How can I be sure I am getting full lecithin value for my dollar?*

ANSWER: Again—be a label reader. Note that lecithin

is obtained solely from soybean oil. Oil contains NO protein. If a lecithin product says it has a protein or amino acid content—it cannot be pure lecithin but contains additives.

QUESTION: *How can I home test my lecithin granule product to make certain it is pure?*

ANSWER: Pure or real lecithin granules disperse rapidly in liquids. Soy flour sinks right to the bottom of a liquid; it is not a natural emulsifier and does NOT dissolve. Test your granules and see what happens.

QUESTION: *Are any tablets available that contain large amounts of choline?*

ANSWER: All tablets providing more than a few milligrams of choline contain one of the synthetic choline compounds: usually choline bitartrate, choline chloride or choline dihydrogen citrate. They do NOT contain phosphatidyl choline, the naturally-occurring dietary source of choline. So you will have to do with the current product of moderate (but very effective) amounts of choline. Purer and more potent phosphatidyl choline preparations do exist, but they are very expensive and usually available solely to the medical and scientific communities.

QUESTION: *How can a label tell me that the potency is higher than usual?*

ANSWER: Read ingredients on a label. Look for the important words "soy phosphatides." This tells you that the product is pure lecithin granules. The higher the percentage of soy phosphatides, the higher the potency and the purer the product!

QUESTION: *What if a product lists choline chloride on the label?*

ANSWER: It's synthetic choline and considered inferior to phosphatidyl choline.

QUESTION: *How natural are choline supplements?*

ANSWER: If such a supplement is either capsule or tablet, it is usually synthetic. Again, read the label and look for the words "pure" or "natural." If in doubt, ask the storekeeper. If you do not receive a satisfactory reply, write to the manufacturer.

QUESTION: *How can lecithin be of help in reducing or eliminating gallstones?*

ANSWER: Scientists suggest that the basic cause of gallstone formation is in the composition of bile (the cholesterol-containing digestive juice that is produced by the liver). Bile is necessary since it helps in bodily absorption of fats. But if metabolism of bile is faulty, cholesterol leaks out of it and forms painful gallstones. Australian doctors have found that by giving gallstone patients lecithin together with cholic acid (a naturally occurring bile substance), there was either a shrinking or dissolution of the gallstones. Furthermore, in three patients, they disappeared completely. The doctors report, "A combination of soybean lecithin and cholic acid does lower the cholesterol saturation of bile and may promote gallstone dissolution." (*Lancet*, December 6, 1975.)

QUESTION: *Is lecithin alone helpful in easing gallstone distress?*

ANSWER: In a study of eight gallstone patients, lecithin was administered alone. Doctors say this food reduced pain and altered bile metabolism in a way that would help dissolve the stones. One lecithin-taking patient had fewer and less serious pain attacks; he showed improved bile chemistry. The size of his gallstones were reduced. This suggests that in some situations, lecithin may be able to correct the problem. (*American Journal of Gastroenterology*, March 1976.)

QUESTION: *What other ailments have been eased with the use of lecithin?*

ANSWER: Let's take them individually, as follows.

Huntington's chorea. It killed famed folk singer-composer Woody Guthrie. It is characterized by jerky involuntary movements and progressive mental deterioration. Doctors who have administered oral doses of choline (from 10 to 20 grams daily) tell us there was marked improvement of the involuntary movements in many such patients. Lecithin is a powerhouse of choline.

Friedrich's ataxia. In this condition, there is speech impairment, lateral curvature of the spine, irregular motions and paralysis. Dr. Andre Barbeau at the University of Montreal treated such patients for just two months with daily doses of lecithin up to 24 grams. Dr. Barbeau says there was an average of "30 percent improvement in speech, balance and movement."

Alzheimer's disease. A tragic mind-destroying ailment which begins sneakily with memory difficulties and renders the patient helpless and almost invalid. From Edinburgh, reports have appeared by Janice Christie, M.D., to the effect that choline supplements are able to delay the insidious progress of body-mind destruction. Similar controls have been established with the use of lecithin by Dr. Pierre Etienne and his medical team at the Allan Memorial Institute in Quebec.

Myasthenia gravis. A form of progressive paralysis. It took the life of Aristotle Onassis. Specifically, it is a defect of transmission across the gap between nerve and muscle. It affects voluntary muscles, weakening them. The muscle fails to respond to stimulation by the trance of acetyl choline released from its controlling nerve, almost as if poisoned. What is needed is an increase of acetyl choline to restore a normal response. This was noted by Adelle Davis in *Let's Get Well:* "A lack of choline itself causes a marked underproduction of acetylcholine and results in muscle weakness, damage to the muscle fibers and extensive scarring. It is accompanied by the urinary loss of a substance, creatine, which invariably shows that the muscles are being destroyed." Therefore, she suggests intake of choline, together with vitamin E because it increases the release and utilization of acetylcholine.

Tardive dyskinesia (or TD). A condition in which the person endures involuntary movements, typically of the mouth area. It is a neurological disorder characterized by bizarre involuntary facial grimaces and body jerking. A team of physicians headed by John H. Growdon, M.D., Alan J. Gelenberg, M.D., and Richard J. Wurtman, M.D. gave lecithin to such troubled patients. Symptoms included tongue protrusions, jaw-chewing motions, lip-puckering movements. The doctors reported there was a satisfactory suppression of these TD symptoms in a good number of these patients. The doctors say they gave choline chloride (synthetic) to some patients and lecithin granules (pure) to others. Results with pure lecithin were more favorable. This substance "may be more acceptable to patients, since it does not have the bitter taste or fishy odor associated with choline (synthetic) ingestion. These data suggest that lecithin may constitute an effective mode of neurotransmitter precursor therapy for conditions in which physicians wish to increase cholinergic tone." (*New England Journal of Medicine*, Vol. 298, No. 18.)

Gallstones. We covered this above but can offer another lecithin healer. David A. Dreiling, M.D., of Mt. Sinai School of Medicine in New York treated gallstone patients with lecithin. He prescribed 0.3 grams of lecithin a day (one tablespoon has 7.5 grams). Yet this small amount (combined with medication) "did result in a more rapid dissolution of stones, perhaps in a shorter interval and at a lower dosage" of the medication. Back in 1965, Adelle Davis also suggested that "a high lecithin content of bile would appear to be vitally important in preventing stones." And coming full circle, we read of reports in the Soviet Union telling that in gallstone patients who were given lecithin daily bile became altered so that there was less of a risk of gallstone formation.

Bleeding problems. A patient troubled with bleeding was treated with an extract of soybeans (presumably, lecithin) by Armand J. Quick, M.D., of the Medical College of Wisconsin. His bleeding time was dangerously high during the twenty-one years he had been treated by the doctor. In a few weeks of lecithin treatment, the bleeding time became normal. Dr. Quick tried the lecithin treatment on another patient and the results were now "even more striking." He continues using lecithin on other people with the same bleeding problem . . . and with the same good results.

And so, lecithin continues to play the leading role in the drama of healthful living. It may well prove to be the nutrition discovery of the century.

8 Using Lecithin for Beauty

BUILDING healthy and younger looking skin (and hair, too) is both an inside and outside job. Because a deficiency of vitamin A may cause dryness and scaliness of skin and scalp, it is of interest to note the favorable influence of lecithin's vitamin A on absorption and utilization.

This phospholipid enhances both the absorption and utilization of skin-scalp nourishing vitamin A and carotene.

Even if you're deficient in vitamin A, lecithin appears to make good use of whatever reserves you have so that it acts as a protective agent and guards against total deficiency.

Heals Ezema. So-called "housewives' eczema" was healed with the use of lecithin, as reported during the 1954 meeting of the Southern Medical Association in Atlanta, Georgia, and thereafter reported in *Chemical Week*.

The presence in detergent solutions of soy lecithin in the range of 0.005 to 0.1 percent has been found to afford protection to cell membranes against the action of powerful synthetic detergents.

Lecithin, itself a surface active substance which is

strongly healing on protein surfaces, is not toxic to cells, even in high concentration. It is believed that lecithin blocks the disorganization of the cell membranes and the denaturation of proteins caused by detergents.

Lecithin in cosmetics. It is an ingredient in many skin creams, soaps, shampoos, lotions and a round of other cosmetics and aids for men and women. Its emollient effect (produced alone or through its action upon any other fatty oils present) and its smoothing function on the skin surface have made it most important for the preservation of your skin.

In particular, lecithin exhibits a strong hydrophilic (water absorbing) and lipophilic (fat absorbing) reaction. This means that a lecithin cosmetic or product will help impart both moisture and needed fatty elements for your skin, preventing dryness and premature wrinkling or aging.

This bi-phase reaction (water-fat absorption) helps create healing as well as cellular regeneration. The "acid mantle" of your skin owes its existence, partially at least, to the lower pH resulting from the presence of free fatty acids and phosphoric acid derived from enzyme action on lecithin and associated phospholipids.

NOTE: Lecithin gives protection to cell membranes against the denaturing action of powerful synthetic detergents. Lecithin counteracts the dry and tacky condition of the skin which suggests the removal of lipid (fatty) substances because of prolonged exposure to detergents.

Regular cosmetics contain other fatty materials which are unable to penetrate skin protein components. Not so with the lecithin containing hydrophilic products. These have a deep penetrating action; they exert a remarkable emollient action and penetration through the epidermis.

In soap it is a superfatting agent, producing a mild, creamy effect, stabilizing the lather and exhibiting a penetrating and stimulating action. By reducing the bubble size, it produces an emollient and soothing creamy reaction.

Because lecithin contains fatty acid radicals, it is able to make sudsy cleansing reactions as well as a moisturizing process that would appear to be healing.

It improves the "slip factor" and reduces frictional abrasion. Even if lecithin is added to synthetic detergent milled toilet bars, it eliminates abrasiveness and acts as a fluidizing or plumping up substance.

Helps the skin breathe The rate of skin respiration tends to slow up in later years. With a reduction of oxygen consumption, the skin becomes aged or parched. You need a product that will activate skin respiration. Such a product should contain lecithin. It tends to send much needed oxygen going right into your skin cells. When your skin breathes, your color and texture improves. Lecithin thus gives your skin a "breath of youthful life."

Shampoo. Lecithin appears to be a bridge between oil and water phases. With the removal of the crude soybean oil from lecithin to produce the granules, the fragrance and color are improved as is the affinity for moisture.

With the use of as little as 2 percent of granules (purified, de-oiled phosphatides derived from soybeans) the cosmetic formulator is able to create high performance shampoos (opaque lotion and clear types) with unique hair conditioning action.

These lecithin-containing shampoos combine good manageability of the hair, especially ease of combing and untangling tresses of the hair when wet. The lecithin gives a desirable sheen, offers protection against the stripping and scalp-drying effect of detergents. This purified lecithin is attracted to the protein surfaces of the hair and is deposited as an extremely thin non-greasy film. This helps improve the health of the scalp (which is skin) and your hair.

Note: The purified granules are beneficial in aqueous-alcohol hair setting preparations to help prevent excessive embrittlement when the hair is blown dry after shampooing.

Other products In another important application, lecithin granules added at a level of 2 to 3 percent to mineral oil greatly improves its effectiveness, not only with respect to emollient and conditioning action but also its moisturizing effect as used in lotions, creams and other products. In liquid makeup with pigment where there may be a drying effect on the skin, this tendency is moderated by including a small percentage of lecithin.

Since lecithin is a vital constituent of billions of your cells and plays a decisive role in cellular metabolism, it follows on theoretical grounds that it would be a desirable ingredient of cosmetic preparations. Skin creams made with even a small percentage of lecithin exhibit greater softening and penetrating benefits.

Those so-called "wrinkle" creams have been compounded with rather high percentages of lecithin. More highly purified or blended grades are desired for use in cosmetics and soap products.

USING LECITHIN AT HOME FOR SKIN HEALTH

Basic formula: To one-quarter cup of water, add one tablespoon of lecithin granules. Blenderize for just two minutes, or until it is of a liquid consistency. This is your *Basic Formula*. Now you may make any of these skin rejuvenating tonics at home.

Skin toner facial. Clean your face well. Rub with egg white and a bit of the Basic Formula. It will tighten on your skin and require plenty of rinsing, but it leaves your complexion rosy, glowing, youthful.

Enlarged pores. Make a paste of oatmeal or cornmeal by mixing with a little water. Add some Basic Formula. Spread on your face and leave for at least fifteen minutes. Rinse with warm water and then cool water.

Oily skin. Avocado blended to a paste with some Basic Formula is great for oily skin. Just let remain for thirty minutes, then splash off.

Dry Skin. Rub your face lightly with olive oil combined with some Basic Formula. Or, mix the juice of a honeydew melon with the Basic Formula and spread on your face.

Lecithin moisturizer

> ½ cup unsaturated oil
> 2 tablespoons anhydrous lanolin (pharmacist or herbalist)
> 3 ounces witch hazel
> 1 tablespoon Basic Formula

Heat water and oil and lanolin. After lanolin has melted and blended with the oil, add the witch hazel and Basic Formula. The mixture should now be warm enough to thicken as you beat it. Quickly remove from heat. Beat to desired consistency.

How to Use: Clean your face and neck thoroughly. Splash warm water over this area. Now gently dip fingertips into this Lecithin Moisturizer and spread cream over the entire area. Let remain about five minutes. Splash off with cold water and gently tissue off. Then use your usual foundation lotion or makeup. (If makeup products have lecithin, so much the better.)

Scalp and hair Your hair is probably your most valuable beauty asset. The plainest person looks great with wonderfully shiny, glossy, fragrant hair. Poets have called it the "crowning glory" . . . and it is just that!

Your weekly shampoo and daily brushing are your most basic hair treatments. Whether you have problem hair or naturally beautiful hair, brushing daily will make it more shiny and healthy right back to your roots. A hundred strokes a day will do it and it is well worth the time. Good exercise, too.

You Will Need: The same Basic Formula as described above.

For Blondes. Rinse your hair in a brew made of one-half cup of camomile flowers, one tablespoon of Basic Formula and two cups of hot water.

For Brunettes. Try a brew of rosemary steeped in water and drained. Add some Basic Formula. Makes for great highlights and sheen.

For Oily Hair. Beat two egg whites with some Basic Formula until stiff. Apply to your scalp with an old toothbrush. Let dry. Brush thoroughly *first* and shampoo afterwards.

For Dry, Lifeless Hair. Rub a combo of castor oil and Basic Formula into your scalp at bedtime. Shampoo in the morning. (Reserve an old pillowcase for oil-treatment use.) Treat twice a week for a few weeks, then once every two weeks. It will make your hair shiny and more healthy. If you don't want to leave the oil on all night, rub castor oil plus Basic formula well into your scalp. Steam it in by pressing a hot towel on your head. Shampoo well.

Dandruff. It can be a nuisance, and stubborn at that. Try mixing equal amounts of vinegar-water-Basic Formula. Part your hair and apply well to your scalp with cotton. Shampoo off.

Shampoo. Beat one raw egg lightly together with Basic Formula, using a fork. Rinse well with warm water.

Super-Shampoo. Buy a bar of castile soap. Cut off slivers with a knife. Cover the shavings with water; add Basic Formula. Simmer over low heat until the soap is melted. Add the amount of water needed for the thickness you desire.

Setting Lotion. Try ordinary milk plus lecithin, instead. It adds body and lustre to your hair, nourishes your scalp and leaves no flakiness or odor. After a shampoo and rinse, spray on a milk plus Basic Formula combo with an atomizer. Comb it through your hair, and set as usual.

With the use of lecithin, inside and outside, you should be able to help yourself look both youthful and healthy.

9 Your Lecithin Cookbook

●▬▬▬◆▬◆▬▬◆▬◆▬▬●

HERE IS a collection of tasty recipes that use lecithin and/or soybeans as one of the ingredients. Plan to use these recipes regularly. You'll help improve your health and enjoy delicious meals at the same time. What more could you ask?

Breakfast

CREAMED BREAKFAST RICE

2 cups cooked brown rice
¾ cup sun-dried raisins

1½ cups milk
2 tablespoons lecithin granules

Mix all ingredients. Pour into deep casserole dish. Cover. Bake at 325°F. for 45 minutes. Do not let milk boil or it will curdle.

SWEDISH RYE MUSH

⅔ cups rye flour
2 tablespoons lecithin granules

3 cups lukewarm water
½ cup sun-dried raisins

Mix rye flour and lecithin into luke warm water. Keep whipping until mixture has no lumps. Stir rapidly as it cooks over a high flame. When it starts to boil, turn heat to low. Cook for 10 minutes, stirring occasionally. Add raisins (or chopped dates) just before taking from stove. This mush thickens even after removing from stove.

ROLLED OAT CEREAL

1 cup rolled oats
2 tablespoons lecithin granules

½ cup ground sunflower seeds
3 cups boiling water

Mix oats and lecithin and sunflower seeds together. Stir into boiling water. Cover. Cook over low heat for 5 minutes.

CRACKED WHEAT CEREAL

1 cup cracked wheat
2 tablespoons lecithin granules

4 cups boiling water

Boil wheat and lecithin in water about 1 hour or in double boiler until soft.

ROLLED OAT WAFFLES

2 cups rolled oats
3 tablespoons lecithin granules

¼ cup vegetable oil
1½ cups milk

Mix all together while waffle iron is heating. Have waffle iron very hot. Let mixture stand about 10 minutes, then spoon into waffle iron using large mixing spoon. These waffles will be crisp and golden brown when done. Waffles are lighter if batter is refrigerated overnight.

SCRAMBLED EGGS

6 eggs
⅓ cup milk
½ cup soybean mash, packed

½ teaspoon salt substitute
2 tablespoons butter or margarine

Beat eggs until frothy. Add milk, soybean mash and salt substitute. Stir well. Melt butter in skillet. Add egg mixture. Cook slowly, stirring gently. Cook until eggs are set but not dry. Serves 6.

Breads

RAISED MUFFINS

2 packages dry yeast
1⅓ cups warm water
1½ teaspoons salt substitute
⅓ cup whole grain flour (gluten flour is good)

1 tablespoon vegetable oil
½ cup molasses
1½ cups unbleached flour
4 tablespoons lecithin granules

Dissolve yeast in ½ cup of the water. Add rest of the water. Stir in all other ingredients lightly. Drop by spoonfuls into well oiled muffin tins. Let raise until twice the size of dough. Bake at 425°F. for 20 minutes.

OATMEAL BREAD

2 cups boiling water
2 cups oatmeal
6 tablespoons lecithin granules
2 packages dry yeast

½ cup lukewarm water
½ cup molasses
½ cup wheat germ
5 cups whole wheat flour

Add boiling water to oatmeal and lecithin. Let stand 1 hour. Dissolve yeast in warm water. Add to oats. Mix in other ingredients. Knead in enough flour to make a smooth dough. Place in oiled pan. Cover. Let rise. Knead down. Cover. Let rise. Oil bread tins and form into loaves. Cover loaves. Let rise. Bake at 375°F. for 1 hour or until they lift out of pans easily.

BOSTON BROWN BREAD

1¾ cups milk
1 package dry yeast
¾ cup molasses
¾ cup sun-dried raisins

1 cup rye meal
1 cup corn meal
1 cup whole wheat flour
4 tablespoons lecithin

Put milk, yeast, molasses and raisins into a mixing bowl. Add sifted flours and lecithin gradually, beating them into the other ingredients. Turn into a well-greased mold. A tall fruit can will do if you do not have a regular mold. Tie cover on securely and steam in hot water for 2 to 3 hours.

SOY BREAD

6 tablespoons lecithin	2½ cups warm water
2 tablespoons honey	2 yeast cakes
2 tablespoons vegetable oil	2 cups unbleached flour
1 tablespoon salt substitute	1½ cups soy flour

Put everything but the flours into a mixing bowl. Dissolve the yeast and stir in the soy and unbleached flours. Turn out on board and knead well. Place in an oiled bowl and cover. Let rise until double its size. Return to board and knead well. Place in a bowl. Cover and let rise until double its size. Form into loaves. Let rise until double in size. Bake at 350°F. for 1 hour. Makes two large loaves or three small ones.

Soups

CREAM OF MUSHROOM SOUP

2 cups minced mushroom (fresh preferred)	2 cups water
1 cup minced celery	½ teaspoon salt substitute
½ cup minced onion	¼ cup minced parsley
2 tablespoons vegetable oil	½ teaspoon brewer's yeast
2 tablespoons water	2 tablespoons lecithin granules
2 tablespoons unbleached flour	2 cups milk

Sauté mushrooms, celery and onions in oil and 2 tablespoons water. Separately, mix flour and water. Turn mushroom combo into sauce pan and add flour and water. Turn heat low and cook slowly. Add salt, parsley, yeast and lecithin granules. Cook and stir for about 15 minutes, then add milk. Reheat, but do not boil. Serve promptly.

SOY CORN CHOWDER

2 cups cooked green soybeans
2 cups diced potatoes
½ cup chopped green onions
1 cup water
2 cups cream style corn

1 cup stewed tomatoes,
2 tablespoons lecithin granules
1 tablespoon vegetable oil
2 cups milk

Cook soybeans, potatoes and onions in water. When these vegetables are tender, add corn, tomatoes, lecithin and vegetable oil. When hot enough to boil, turn off heat. Add warm milk and serve.

VEGETABLE BROTH

3 cups finely chopped celery
3 cups grated carrots
1 cup chopped spinach
1 cup parsley, chopped fine

¼ cup green onion, chopped fine
2 tablespoons lecithin granules
Optional: 1 cup tomato juice

Simmer in 2 quarts of water for 15 to 20 minutes. Strain. *Suggestion:* add 1 cup tomato juice, if desired. Delicious served hot or cold.

MINERAL BROTH

2 medium potatoes, scrubbed well, cut in small wedges
1 cup parsley, chopped fine
4 green onions, chopped fine
4 stalks of celery, leaves and all

2 carrots, scrubbed well and cut in small pieces
1 cup chopped chard (or turnip tops or mustard tops)
3 tablespoons lecithin granules

Simmer slowly. Season with salt substitute.

HEALTH SOUP

5 medium tomatoes
½ large ripe avocado
1 cup carrot juice
½ teaspoon onion powder

Pinch garlic powder
1 cup celery juice
3 tablespoons lecithin granules

Put tomatoes and avocado in blender and liquefy. Add all remaining ingredients. Pour into double boiler. Heat until hot but do not boil. *Suggestion*: Add 2 teaspoons chopped parsley. Serve promptly.

SOYBEAN VEGETABLE SOUP

1 cup dry soybeans
6½ cups water
2 ounces beef chunks
1 16-ounce can tomatoes
1 cup celery, sliced
1 cup carrots, diced

½ cup turnips, diced
½ cup onion, sliced
3 beef bouillon cubes
⅛ teaspoon garlic powder
1 bay leaf
Salt substitute to taste

Soak soybeans overnight in 3 cups water. Discard soaking water. Now add remaining 3½ cups water and meat to beans; cover and cook slowly for 2 hours. Add vegetables and seasonings. Cover and cook slowly 35 minutes until vegetables are tender and flavors blended. Remove bay leaf before serving. Serves 6.

SPANISH LENTIL SOUP

1 cup cooked lentils	1 tablespoon vegetable oil
2 cups chopped green onions	3 tablespoons lemon juice
2 quarts cold water	3 tablespoons lecithin granules
1 tablespoon salt substitute	
¼ cup chopped sweet green peppers	2 cups chopped raw spinach

Combine all ingredients, except spinach, in large kettle. Cook until soft. Now add spinach. Cook 10 minutes longer.

Vegetables

Soybeans may be enjoyed simply by seasoning with butter or margarine and serving as a vegetable or in favorite recipes in place of lima beans.

BAKED ZUCCHINI SQUASH

To Begin: Parboil the long green squash until they are almost done, but still hold their shape. Split lengthwise, scoop out center. Chop this center. Mix with following ingredients and stuff into squash shells.

2 cups bean sprouts	2 tablespoons vegetable oil
4 chopped green onions	1 teaspoon salt
2 stalks of celery, chopped	2 tablespoons lecithin granules
1 cup sliced mushrooms	

Bake at 425°F. until light brown, so that the bean sprouts are tender but not mushy.

BAKED EGGPLANT

To Begin: Peel and slice eggplant and soak in water.

Meantime mix:

1 cup wheat germ or bran or combo	2 tablespoons lecithin granules
½ cup brewer's yeast flakes	1 tablespoon onion powder
	1 cup milk

Now roll drained eggplant in this mixture. Carefully lay into a deep, well-oiled baking dish, and pour milk over eggplant slices. Cover. Bake at 425°F. for 1 hour.

FRESH SUCCOTASH

2 cups cooked soybeans	½ cup milk
1 cup cold water	2 tablespoons lecithin granules
2 cups fresh corn kernels	

Cook beans in saucepan; add corn. Cook five minutes. Water should be almost gone. Add milk and lecithin. Reheat but do not boil. Serve promptly.

PEAS WITH MUSHROOMS

4 cups fresh peas
½ cup water
1 cup sliced fresh mushrooms

1 tablespoons chopped parsley
2 tablespoons lecithin granules

Cook together in heavy tight-lidded sauce pan for 15 to 20 minutes.

SOYBEAN-CORN-TOMATO CASSEROLE

2½ cups dry soybeans, cooked and drained
1 16-ounce can whole-kernel corn, drained
1 16-ounce can tomatoes
2 tablespoons soy flour
1 teaspoon garlic powder

¼ teaspoon basil leaves, crushed
1 cup bran or wheat germ (or combo)
½ cup Cheddar cheese, shredded
2 tablespoons butter or margarine

Preheat oven to 375°F. (moderate).

Arrange beans and corn in alternate layers in a 2-quart baking dish. Mash tomatoes with a fork; save 2 tablespoons tomato juice. Now mix flour and seasonings; stir into tomato juice. Stir flour mixture into tomatoes. Heat until mixture comes to a boil. Pour hot sauce over vegetables. Mix bran, cheese and butter; sprinkle over vegetables. Bake about 20 minutes until browned. Serves 6.

COLD BEAN SALAD

2 cups cold cooked soybeans
⅔ cup diced celery
¼ cup chopped pickles or well-drained pickle relish
2 tablespoons grated onion
2 teaspoons apple cider vinegar

½ teaspoon salt substitute
¼ to ⅓ cup favorite salad dressing
2 chopped hard-cooked eggs
2 tablespoons chopped green pepper (optional)

Combine all ingredients and mix lightly. Chill in refrigerator at least 1 hour before serving. Serve on lettuce or other salad greens. Serves 4 to 6.

GREEN SOYBEAN SALAD

15-ounce can green soybeans, drained
½ cup celery, finely chopped
1 large tomato, diced
¼ cup green pepper, chopped

Favorite French dressing
¼ teaspoon salt substitute
Lettuce or salad greens, several leaves

Mix all ingredients except lettuce. Toss lightly. Chill thoroughly to blend flavors. Serve on lettuce. Serves 4 to 6.

LEMON SOYBEAN SPROUTS

5 cups soybean sprouts
3 cups boiling water
1½ teaspoons salt substitute
2 tablespoons butter or margarine

1 tablespoon arrowroot powder
1 tablespoon fresh lemon juice

Cook sprouts in boiling salted water 10 to 15 minutes until just tender. Drain sprouts, saving 1 cup liquid. Add butter to hot vegetable liquid. Mix arrowroot powder and lemon juice and add to vegetable liquid; cook and stir until thickened. Add sprouts and pepper. Heat to serving temperature. Serves 4 to 6.

Main Courses

PEANUT BUTTER LOAF

2 cups grated raw carrots
1 cup cooked brown rice
½ cup shelled peanuts, chopped fine
½ cup bran
3 tablespoons chopped onion

1 cup milk
3 tablespoons oil
⅛ teaspoon sage
3 tablespoons lecithin granules

Mix together. Cover and let stand about 30 minutes. Pour into oiled baking dish. Cover and bake for 60 minutes at 350°F.

WALNUT ROAST

1 medium onion, chopped fine
2 tablespoons vegetable oil
1½ cups milk
1½ cups wheat germ or bran or combo

1 cup ground walnuts
1 teaspoon salt substitute
2 tablespoons parsley, chopped fine
4 tablespoons lecithin granules

Sauté onions in oil. Mix in all remaining ingredients.

Let stand 30 minutes, covered. Turn into an oiled baking dish. Bake for 60 minutes at 350°F.

SUNFLOWER LOAF

1 cup ground walnuts
½ cup wheat germ or bran or combo
½ cup grated raw potato
1 cup milk
3 tablespoons grated onion
½ cup ground sunflower seeds
3 tablespoons lecithin granules
1 tablespoon oil

Mix well. Let stand, covered, for 30 minutes. Bake at 350°F. for 60 minutes.

LECITHIN BURGERS

½ cup walnuts
1 medium small raw potato
1 cup cooked oatmeal
4 tablespoons vegetable oil
1 cup toasted wheat germ
4 tablespoons lecithin granules
⅓ teaspoon sage
1 teaspoon brewer's yeast powder
1 teaspoon soy flour
Enough soy milk to moisten

Grind nuts and potato. Add all other ingredients, dissolving the yeast in ¼ cup hot water. Add enough soy milk to moisten ingredients, then cover and set aside for 30 minutes. Form into patties. Broil, braise or sauté in very little oil until golden brown.

MEAT LOAF

1 cup bran or wheat germ (or combo)
2 tablespoons minced onion
¾ cup milk
2 eggs, beaten
1 teaspoon salt substitute

1¼ pounds ground beef
½ cup soybean mash, packed
¼ cup tomato puree
1 teaspoon Worcestershire sauce

Preheat oven to 350°F. (moderate). Soak bran and onion in milk until soft. Stir in eggs, salt substitute. Gently mix in ground beef and soybean mash. Press into a baking pan, about 9 × 5 inches. Bake just 1 hour. Meantime, mix tomato puree and Worcestershire sauce. Set aside. Remove loaf from oven. Drain off fat. Spread tomato mixture over meat loaf. Bake 10 minutes longer. Cool slightly before slicing. Serves 6.

LECITHIN LOAF

1 cup pureed cooked lima beans
1 cup grated coconut
3 tablespoons grated onion
2 teaspoons vegetable oil

1 cup lecithin granules
2 cups cooked brown rice
½ cup chopped parsley
Optional: pinch of thyme

Mix all ingredients together and turn into oiled baking dish. Bake at 450°F. for 20 minutes, then lower to 350°F. for 40 minutes. Serve with brown gravy.

CARROT-RICE-LECITHIN LOAF

½ cup natural peanut butter
1 cup milk
2 cups grated carrots
1 cup cold cooked brown rice
2 teaspoons grated onion

½ cup wheat germ or bran or combo
3 tablespoons vegetable oil
½ teaspoon sage, or to taste
4 tablespoons lecithin granules

Mix milk and peanut butter to a smooth paste; add all other ingredients. Bake at 325°F. for 60 minutes in oiled baking dish.

LECITHIN-STUFFED PEPPERS

4 green peppers
2 cups mashed cooked soybeans
½ cup finely chopped celery
½ cup finely shredded carrots

4 tablespoons lecithin granules
¼ cup minced onion
½ cup finely chopped walnuts
¼ cup tomato sauce or tomato pulp

Remove seeds and partitions from inside of green peppers. Boil 3 minutes, drain. Fill with mixture of all ingredients and bake 30 minutes at 325°F. or until peppers are soft.

OATMEAL PATTIES

1 raw potato, medium size
½ cup nuts
4 green onions, chopped fine
4 tablespoons vegetable oil

1 cup cooked oatmeal
4 tablespoons lecithin granules
1 tablespoon chopped parsley

Grind potato and nuts. Simmer potato and onion in oil until soft. Mix with oatmeal, nuts, and remaining ingredients. Form into patties. Bake at 350°F. on oiled cookie sheet or saute lightly.

LECITHIN ROAST

2 cups lima beans, cooked and mashed
1 cup cooked millet
½ cup lecithin granules
½ cup ground nuts

⅓ cup chopped green onion
⅓ cup celery
2 tablespoons parsley, cut fine
⅓ cup grated carrots
½ cup milk

Mix all together, adding milk last, a little at a time, until mixture is the right consistency for roast. Bake at 375°F. in an oiled pan, for 60 minutes.

LENTIL-LECITHIN PATTIES

3 tablespoons chopped green onion
2 tablespoons vegetable oil
2 cups cooked mashed lentils

3 cups mashed potato
½ cup lecithin granules
½ teaspoon chopped parsley
Salt substitute to taste

Soften onion in oil over low heat. Put remaining ingredients in bowl. Add onions and oil. Stir mixture. Form into patties. Brown lightly on oiled skillet.

Desserts

APPLE CRISP

4 cups sliced apples
½ cup honey
¼ teaspoon cinnamon

⅔ cup soy flour (any type)
¼ cup butter

Combine sliced apples, honey and cinnamon and place in a well-greased 8 × 8 × 2 inch pan. Work flour in butter until a crumbly mixture is formed. Sprinkle this mixture over the apples. Bake in a hot oven (400°F.) for 20 to 25 minutes. Serves 6 to 8.

APPLESAUCE CAKE

1 cup butter or margarine
1¾ cups honey
2 beaten eggs
1½ cups thick applesauce
2½ teaspoons baking powder
½ teaspoon nutmeg

¾ teaspoon baking soda
1 cup soy flour
2½ cups sifted flour, whole grain
1 teaspoon salt substitute

Cream butter with honey, add beaten eggs and applesauce. Sift all other ingredients together and stir into the first mixture. Pour into a well-greased 9 × 13 inch pan. Bake in a slow oven (325°F.) for 1 hour. NOTE: This cake may be made several days ahead, as the flavor improves with age. Serves 4 to 6.

PLAN TO ENJOY LECITHIN DAILY

Use the preceding recipes as a tasty way to lecithin-nourish your body and mind every single day as well as using soy lecithin granules as a supplement. Lecithin can regenerate your total being.

The Best in Health Books by
LINDA CLARK,
BEATRICE TRUM HUNTER
and CARLSON WADE

By Linda Clark

☐ **Know Your Nutrition**   Paperback $3.50
☐ **Face Improvement Through Nutrition** $2.25
☐ **Be Slim and Healthy** $1.50
☐ **Go-Caution-Stop Carbohydrate Computer** $1.25
☐ **Light on Your Health Problems** $1.50
☐ **The Best of Linda Clark** $3.50
☐ **How to Improve Your Health**   Paperback $4.95

By Beatrice Trum Hunter

☐ **Whole Grain Baking Sampler**
   ☐ **Cloth $6.95**   ☐ **Paperback $2.95**
☐ **Food Additives and Your Health** $2.25
☐ **Fermented Foods and Beverages** $1.25
☐ **Yogurt, Kefir & Other Milk Cultures** $1.75
☐ **Food and Your Health** (Anthology ed. by BTH) $1.50

By Carlson Wade

☐ **Arthritis and Nutrition** $1.95
☐ **Bee Pollen** $2.25
☐ **Lecithin** $2.25
☐ **Fats, Oils and Cholesterol** $1.50
☐ **Vitamins and Other Supplements** $1.25
☐ **Hypertension (High Blood Pressure)** $1.50
  and Your Diet

Buy them at your local health or book store or use this coupon.

COOKBOOKS ON NATURAL HEALTH
... To Help You Eat Better for Less!

☐ **ADD A FEW SPROUTS** (Martha H. Oliver)	**$1.95**
☐ **WHOLE GRAIN BAKING SAMPLER** (Beatrice Trum Hunter)	**$2.95**
☐ **MRS. APPLEYARD'S KITCHEN** (L.A. Kent)	**$3.95**
☐ **MRS. APPLEYARD'S SUMMER KITCHEN** (L.A. Kent & E.K. Gay)	**$3.95**
☐ **MRS. APPLEYARD'S WINTER KITCHEN** (L.A. Kent & E.K. Gay)	**$3.95**
☐ **BETTER FOODS FOR BETTER BABIES** (Gena Larson)	**$1.75**
☐ **GOOD FOODS THAT GO TOGETHER** (Esther L. Smith)	**$3.95**
☐ **MEALS AND MENUS FOR ALL SEASONS** (Agnes Toms)	**$1.25**
☐ **NATURAL FOODS BLENDER COOKBOOK** (Frieda Nusz)	**$1.95**
☐ **BONNIE FISHER'S WAY WITH HERBS**	**$2.95**
☐ **GOOD FOOD, GLUTEN FREE** (Hilda Cherry Hills)	**$3.50**
☐ **LOAVES AND FISHES** (Malvina Kinard & Janet Crisler)	**$4.95**
☐ **MENNONITE COMMUNITY COOKBOOK** (Mary Emma Showalter)	**$1.25**
☐ **EAT THE WEEDS** (Ben Charles Harris)	**$1.50**

Buy them at your local health or book store or use this coupon.

- -

Keats Publishing, Inc. (P.O. Box 876), New Canaan, Conn. 06840 75-G
Please send me the books I have checked above. I am enclosing
$_____ (add 50¢ to cover postage and handling). Send check or
money order — no cash or C.O.D.'s please.

Mr/Mrs/Miss_____

Address _____

City _____ State _____ Zip _____
(Allow three weeks for delivery.)